Back Stability

Christopher M. Norris, MSc, MCSP
Director, Norris Associates, Manchester, UK

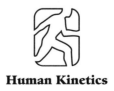

Human Kinetics

Library of Congress Cataloging-In-Publication Data

Norris, Christopher M.
    Back stability / Christopher M. Norris.
        p. cm.
    Includes bibliographical references and index.
    ISBN 0-7360-0081-X
    1. Backache--Treatment. 2. Backache--Prevention. 3. Backache--Exercise therapy. I.
Title.

RD771.I58 N67 2000
617.5'64--dc21   99-089545

ISBN 0-7360-0081-X

Permission notices for material reprinted in this book from other sources can be found on
page 263.

Acquisitions Editor: Loarn D. Robertson, PhD; **Developmental Editor**: Elaine Mustain;
Writer: Brian Mustain; **Assistant Editors**: Derek Campbell, Melissa Feld, Maggie Schwarzen-
traub; **Copyeditor**: Lisa Morgan; **Proofreader**: Myla Smith; **Indexer**: Craig Brown; **Permission Manager**: Heather Munson; **Graphic Designer**: Fred Starbird; **Graphic Artist**: Yvonne
Griffith; **Cover Designer**: Keith Blomberg; **Photographer (cover)**: Tom Roberts; **Art Manager**: Craig Newsom; **Illustrator**: Kristin Mount; **Printer**: Edwards Brothers

Printed in the United States of America   10 9 8 7 6 5 4 3

Human Kinetics
Web site: www.HumanKinetics.com

United States: Human Kinetics
P.O. Box 5076
Champaign, IL 61825-5076
800-747-4457
e-mail: humank@hkusa.com

Canada: Human Kinetics
475 Devonshire Road, Unit 100
Windsor, ON N8Y 2L5
800-465-7301 (in Canada only)
e-mail: orders@hkcanada.com

Europe: Human Kinetics
107 Bradford Road
Stanningley
Leeds LS28 6AT, United Kingdom
+44 (0)113 255 5665
e-mail: hk@hkeurope.com

Australia: Human Kinetics
57A Price Avenue
Lower Mitcham, South Australia 5062
08 8277 1555
e-mail: liahka@senet.com.au

New Zealand: Human Kinetics
P.O. Box 105-231, Auckland Central
09-523-3462
e-mail: hkp@ihug.co.nz

Contents

Part IV ▪ Putting It All Together   229

Preface

This book presents an approach to treating low back pain that is different from what you've seen before. I'd like to present a brief story to illustrate my point. One of the editorial staff who worked on this book had experienced severe back problems for over a quarter century. Only a few months before he saw this manuscript, he had completed a 12-week intensive weight-training program that he had hoped would help his back. It provided some relief, but not a great deal. After he had read the manuscript, this person began employing just a couple of the very elementary principles described in chapter 4 (specifically, hollowing his abdomen and intentionally tightening his multifidus muscles). He did not even do any of the exercises—he just practiced abdominal hollowing and multifidus tightening as he sat at his desk, or in his car, or as he walked through the supermarket. A month after he began this *very* minimal effort, he reported to me that his sharp sciatica pain had declined about 80% and that his periodic minor (but quite distressing) bowel incontinence, caused by impingement of vertebrae on a nerve, had declined from about a dozen episodes per week to about one every two weeks.

While I certainly do *not* endorse this person's decision to do only the bare minimum in trying to alleviate his back problems, I note the story here to illustrate a single point: *This approach works!*

It works because it is based on sound anatomical, physiological, and neurological principles. While health professionals have long known that a large number of back problems arise because of muscle weakness, solving the problems simply by "doing strengthening exercises" is like telling a person with an infection to "take a lot of antibiotics" without targeting the medicine to the microbe.

I have treated scores of "hunks" who had terrible problems with lower back pain. An individual can have unusually strong abdominal and back muscles while those unsung, unpublicized, invisible muscles that run alongside the spine—and that actually keep it stable—are weak and stretched. This book shows you how to help your clients solve lower back problems *by attending to the actual anatomical structures that control the problem*—and these are *not* merely the gross, obvious muscles that make one look good at the beach. They are nearly invisible muscles such as the transversus abdominis and the multifidus; invisible tendons that have become inelastic; and hidden nerves carrying invisible impulses, all of which can be trained surprisingly well (I'll teach you how) to stabilize the back even when your client isn't thinking about it. I have honed the techniques described in this book over many years, during which I have helped thousands of clients who for the most part had not been significantly helped with traditional approaches.

If you ever treat, advise, coach, train, massage, or in any other way deal with people who have lower back pain, this book is for you. If you're a physical therapist, a massage therapist, a chiropractor, an athletic trainer, or a sports physician, this book may well prove vital to your professional practice. Even if you are a casual reader and are not able to understand the more technical aspects, you at least can benefit from learning the basic moves that stabilize the back, as in chapter 4.

Because the body is a complex unit of closely interconnecting systems, any treatment must address the whole, even though it targets a single system. Thus, back stability is part of a holistic approach centering on muscle balance. Muscles affect the support of the spine, posture, and both our ability to move and the way that we move. If we examine the biomechanical factors at work in the back, we can see that there are three elements that combine to restore the muscle balance that is vital to back stability: correction of segmental control, shortening and strengthening lax muscles, and lengthening tight muscles. In *Back Stability*, I will explain these three elements to you, and I'll show you how to order them according to each client's symptoms, using them to construct a program uniquely tailored for that client.

In part I ("The Conceptual Foundation"), I lead you through the anatomical, physiological, and neurological underpinnings of back pain, and of both traditional and newer approaches to treating it. I help you understand *why* traditional approaches so often don't work, and *why* the back stabilization method is so successful. Then, in part II ("Exercises for Establishing Stability"), I show you how to teach your clients the basic skills for back stabilization. In part III ("Building Back Fitness"), I teach you a wide range of exercises that will help your clients prevent recurrence of back pain and rehabilitate their backs (when appropriate) for strenuous on-the-job lifting or for challenging sports activities. Finally, in part IV ("Putting It All Together"), I discuss how you decide which assessments, exercises, etc., to prescribe for which clients. Be sure you don't begin applying the material herein to your clients till after you've studied chapter 10 since that's the roadmap that helps you navigate the exercises with a particular client in mind. Chapter 11, while short, is vital, as it briefly points out how you should coach your clients to avoid reinjuring their backs.

Simple stick figures rather than lifelike line drawings have been used to represent human beings in the illustrations of those exercises in which the position of the pelvic girdle might otherwise be difficult for a layperson to understand. This device makes it easier for your clients to see the required position of the pelvic girdle in those particular exercises. When more life-like drawings were deemed clearer, we have used them. Therefore you, the practitioner, can use the book as a teaching tool, showing your clients the drawings as you explain the exercises to them, and they will be able to see clearly what the desired positions are.

Christopher M. Norris

Acknowledgments

I would like to thank Brian Mustain for translating British English into American English and for unraveling the "knotted ball of wool" that formed my thoughts, and Elaine Mustain for maintaining the book's momentum when all seemed lost.

In addition to the references quoted in this book, I acknowledge the work of several individuals in the field of back stability—including Carolyn Richardson, Gwendolen Jull, Paul Hodges, and Julie Hides from the University of Queensland, Australia; Vladamir Janda and Karl Lewit from the University of Prague, Czech Republic; Shirley Sahrmann from the University of Washington, U.S.A.; and Mark Comerford from Kinetic Control, England.

I would also like to thank the staff at Norris Associates, Manchester, England, for sharing their clinical experience in the field of back stability.

PART

I

The Conceptual
Foundation

Because the approach used in this book differs somewhat from what you have seen in the past, it is important that you understand the theoretical basis for what you read. I begin in chapter 1 ("What Is Back Stability?") with a general introduction to the problems of back pain and back instability. In one sense, the true "problem" is that some health professionals fail to understand that instability IS the problem for many instances of low back pain! People who suffer from back pain may be subjected to manipulation, instructed to perform exercises, told to "work out"; they may be given chemicals to relax their muscles and poked with electric needles—all intended to alleviate their pain. But surprisingly few professionals understand that a great deal of low back pain occurs for one simple reason: the spine is not supported by the tissues surrounding it and therefore "wobbles" in ways that impinge on nerves and in general do bad things to a person's quality of life. Traditional approaches are often quite helpful—but there are some clients for whom they simply do not address the root problem of back pain completely.

The purpose of this book is to teach you how to deal with back pain by helping your clients stabilize their spines. From discussion of the basic etiology of pain in chapter 1, I proceed in chapter 2 ("Biomechanics of the Lumbar Spine") to an explanation of how the spine works: its anatomy, its movements, even the physics of lifting.

Then, in chapter 3 ("Stabilization Mechanisms in the Lumbar Spine"), I show you how the anatomical lessons of the first two chapters lead logically to certain specific, but frequently ignored, treatments.

I hope you will digest these three chapters thoroughly—without their conceptual foundation, the rest of the book will appear to be little more than one more listing of exercises. If you appreciate the anatomical and physiological underpinnings of the following chapters, however, you will see that the "how to" chapters will open for your clients a world of new possibilities that traditional programs cannot provide.

1
What Is
Back Stability?

Back pain is a universal problem, particularly important in the largely sedentary Western world. New information about this condition is stimulating new ways to manage it, focusing particularly on new approaches to exercise.

THE SCOPE OF THE PROBLEM

As many as 80% of individuals in the Western world will suffer at least one disabling episode of low back pain during their lives; at any time, as many as 35% of the population suffers from some kind of back pain (Frymoyer and Cats-Baril 1991). The cost is tremendous, both financially and in terms of personal suffering. Most individuals with low back pain recover within six weeks, but 5-15% of subjects progress to permanent disability, accounting for up to 90% of total expenditures for this condition (Liebenson 1996). Unfortunately, recurrence of back pain after an acute episode is common. Over 60% of individuals suffering an acute episode of low back pain will experience another bout within a year, and 45% of these will have a second recurrence within the following four years (Liebenson 1996).

KEY POINT: As many as 15% of individuals with low back pain progress to permanent disability, and 60% suffer from a recurrence of pain within one year.

Back pain is universal. Sufferers in the United States spend $60 billion per year treating it (Frymoyer and Gordon 1989) and receive $27 billion for permanent disability. The rate of increase in back pain is 14 times greater than the population growth, and during a period when disability awards for all conditions rose by 347%, awards for back pain increased by 2,680% (Frymoyer and Cats-Baril 1991).

In the United Kingdom, 46.5 million working days were lost through back pain in 1989—representing a cost to the National Health Service of £0.5 billion ($840 million) per year and an even larger cost to industry of £5.1 billion ($8.59 billion) in lost production (CSP 1998; Tye and Brown 1990). In 1994-1995, 14 million people in the UK visited their doctors for back pain and lost 116 million working days.

A NEW LOOK AT THE ETIOLOGY AND TREATMENT OF BACK PAIN

In spite of the tremendous increase in the number of back pain sufferers in the past two decades, popular understanding about the nature of back pain has remained somewhat static. It is commonly believed that back pain results from a structural injury or fault that must be corrected in order to reduce pain and restore full function. According to this viewpoint, normal function is impossible—or even dangerous—until the defective *structure* has changed (Zusman 1998).

While it is true that many individuals with low back pain exhibit structural changes, CT (computerized tomography) scans reveal similar "positive findings" in up to 50% of normal, asymptomatic subjects (Boden et al. 1990; Jensel et al. 1994)! It is the same with radiographic changes in the lumbar spine: as many individuals without pain show evidence of disc degeneration as do those with pain (Nachemson 1992). Moreover, studies with cadavers have shown no correlation between structural changes in the lumbar spine and a history of low back pain (Videman et al. 1990), and large disc lesions with nerve compression may be totally asymptomatic (Saal 1995).

KEY POINT: ▷ Structural changes in the spine are as likely in asymptomatic individuals as in those with low back pain and loss of function.

Nonorganic Causes of Back Pain

At least three sources of back pain do not originate in the sufferer's body: iatrogenic, forensic, and behavioral (compare Zusman 1998).

• **Iatrogenic** factors (brought on by the practitioner) include labels of disability and the consequences of deconditioning through prolonged (bed) rest. For example, a label such as "prolapsed disc" is far more threatening to a patient than "simple back pain," even though the total amount of pain experienced by the patient may be the same in both cases. Labels that imply disease or disability such as "arthritis" also suggest severe conditions even though a mild form of the pathology may be present. Alternatives such as "slight roughening" or "normal wear and tear" are less threatening. Although avoiding stressful activities on the back is important, and limited rest has its place, *prolonged* bed rest has been shown to be counterproductive. Deyo et al. (1986) compared two days of bed rest with two weeks of bed rest. They found both periods to be equally effective in terms of pain reduction, but the two-week period led to significant "negative effects due to immobilization" (such as weakening and stiffness around the spine) that were not present in the two-day period.

• **Forensic** factors (associated with legal proceedings) contribute significantly to chronic back pain. In a study of 2,000 back pain patients (Long 1995), involvement in litigation was the only factor that accurately predicted that a person would *not* rapidly return to work.

• Two important **behavioral** factors are perceived disability and anticipation of pain.

1. **Perceived disability.** Patients often fail to take part in daily activities because they *believe* they are physically incapable of doing the task— although structural changes in their spines do not bear out this belief (Zusman 1998). Perceived disability is often associated with a mistaken fear of reinjury (Vlaeyen et al. 1995).

2. **Anticipation of pain.** Often the anticipation of pain rather than pain itself is enough to limit activity and create protective behaviors (Zusman 1998). The physical changes brought about by the fear of pain can be measured on surface EMG (sEMG). Main and Watson (1996) applied experimental noxious stimuli to the upper trapezius on normal subjects and on those with back pain. Normal subjects showed the expected reflex increase in sEMG activity in the trapezius muscles. Those with back pain, however, showed the reaction not in the upper trapezius, but in the lumbar region— suggesting that the subjects viewed any pain *as an inherent part of their back condition* even when the pain was in fact occurring in another part of their bodies.

> **KEY POINT:** Perceived disability and the anticipation of pain contribute significantly to loss of function.

A New Model for Low Back Pain Management

Most people traditionally have perceived back pain as a structural condition that requires rest to recover. New information is challenging this approach, however, viewing back pain at least in part as a functional change that requires functional management. Exercise is at the forefront of this new approach.

The Traditional Model

Rest is still the most common treatment for back pain, despite the fact that prolonged bed rest has been shown to be harmful. Controlled exercises restore function, reduce both distress and perceived disability, diminish pain, and promote a return to work (Waddell 1987). Rest has little effect on the natural history of back pain and may actually increase its severity (Twomey and Taylor 1994). For back pain without significant radiation, bed rest probably should be limited to a maximum of two days. Longer periods are almost certainly counterproductive due to the negative effects of whole-body immobilization (Spitzer et al. 1987).

Surgery is effective in only a small group of low back pain patients. Waddell (1987) argued that surgical intervention can help only 1% of patients. Comparing surgically and conservatively treated patients suffering from disc prolapse, Weber (1983) found no difference in outcome after two years. Aggressive conservative management can successfully treat over 80% of patients with clinically diagnosed sciatica and radiological evidence of nerve root entrapment (Bush et al. 1992). According to Allan and Waddell (1989), "disc surgery . . . [has left] more tragic human wreckage in its wake than any other operation in history."

The New Model

In proposing a new model for the treatment of low back pain, Waddell (1987) recommended that the patient's role should change from one of resting and being a passive recipient of treatment to an active role of sharing responsibility for restoration of function. Rehabilitation professionals increasingly are adopting this philosophy, using exercise programs to enhance lumbar stabilization (Jull and Richardson 1994b; Norris 1995a; O'Sullivan et al. 1997). Here are some examples:

• For a **herniated lumbar disc.** A rehabilitation program that emphasized *skill-based exercise therapy* for the spine effectively treated herniated lumbar discs (Saal and Saal 1989) and rehabilitated football players with back injury (Saal 1988). The program aimed to restore automatic control of muscular stabilization of the trunk by teaching subjects to maintain a correct lumbar pelvic position (i.e., "neutral position"—see following discussion) while performing progressively more complex tasks. In a study by Skall et al. (1994), intensive exercise *when pain was not a limiting factor* was more effective than mild mobilizing exercise five weeks following disc surgery. A one-year follow-up showed a trend favoring the intensive exercise group. Even when the diagnosis is uncertain, progressive exercise—consisting of strengthening, proprioceptive training, and aerobic training—may restore pain-free function (Deutsch 1996). Pain, physical dysfunction, and psychosocial dysfunction improved following a 10-week exercise program for chronic low back pain patients studied by Risch et al. (1993), whereas all three factors worsened for those who remained inactive.

• For **spondylolysis** or **spondylolisthesis**. A back stability program targeting the anterolateral abdominals and multifidus was more effective than conventional rehabilitation in patients with radiographic diagnosis of spondylolysis or spondylolisthesis (O'Sullivan et al. 1997). In this study, one group of patients underwent a 10-week program of gym work (including trunk curl exercises), general exercises such as swimming, and pain-relieving modalities. A second group, which engaged only in back stability exercises, showed a statistically significant reduction in pain intensity, pain descriptor scale, and functional disability that was maintained at a 30-month follow-up (figure 1.1). This trial provides the strongest evidence so far in the literature regarding the effectiveness of stabilization programs for the lumbar spine. I have expanded some of these techniques for use in this book.

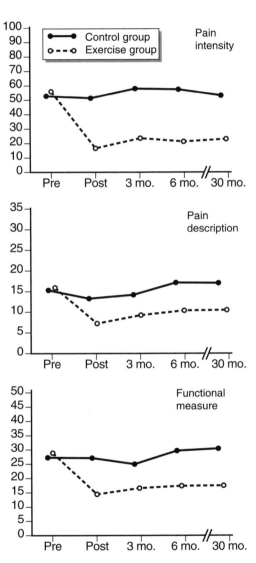

Figure 1.1 A comparison of conventional exercise and stability exercise effects on spondylolysis/spondylolisthesis.

Adapted from O'Sullivan et al. 1997.

THE MODEL USED IN THIS BOOK: LUMBAR STABILIZATION

This book presents a program of back treatment based on the

new model of active patient participation. The most important concept underlying the program is that of lumbar back stability versus lumbar back instability.

Instability of the lumbar spine is not the same as *hypermobility*. In both conditions the range of motion is greater than normal. However, instability is present when there is "an excessive range of abnormal movement for which there is no protective muscular control." There is no instability in hypermobility, however, since the "excessive range of movement . . . has complete muscular control" (Maitland 1986). The essential feature of stability is therefore *the ability of the body to control the whole range of motion of a joint, in this case the lumbar spine.*

> **KEY POINT:** ▸ Stability of a joint implies the body's ability *to control the entire range of motion* around that joint.

An unstable lumbar spine cannot maintain correct vertebral alignment. Because the unstable segment is less stiff (less resistant to movement), movement within the spinal column increases even under minor loads— thereby altering both the quality and quantity of motion. Unstable lumbar spines often reveal no clinical damage to the spinal cord or nerve roots and no incapacitating deformity. If untreated, however, an unstable spine may irritate or damage neural tissue, leading to positive neurological signs on clinical examination. Positive neurological examination therefore does not preclude prescription of stabilization exercise since instability may indeed be the cause of the positive findings.

The excessive movement in an unstable spine may either stretch or compress pain-sensitive structures, leading to inflammation (Kirkaldy-Willis 1990; Panjabi 1992). A number of physical signs can suggest instability in a clinical assessment, as outlined in "Physical Signs of Instability," below. See also "Preliminary Assessment of Your Client," page 231.

Physical Signs of Instability

- Step deformity (spondylolisthesis) or rotation deformity (spondylolisis) on standing, which reduces on lying
- Transverse band of muscle spasm, which reduces on lying
- Localized muscle twitching while shifting weight from one leg to the other
- Juddering or shaking during forward bending
- Alteration to passive intervertebral motion testing, suggesting excessive mobility in the sagittal plane

Source: Paris 1985; Maitland 1986

Stable Movement and Position of the Lumbar Spine

Both the gross and fine positions of the lumbar spine are vital to back stability and may be described in terms of "neutral zone" and "neutral position." Control of these positions requires an interplay among several body systems and forms the basis of the back stability program.

Movement in the Neutral Zone

Lumbar instability may be defined as an excessive range of motion *without* muscular control. Another way to visualize instability is as a loss of stiffness (Pope and Panjabi 1985)—not the negative condition we refer to when we speak of "a stiff back," but rather a positive factor referring to the amount of resistance a structure (in this case, the spine) provides in order to move against a force. (Imagine a bodybuilder arm wrestling a weakling, and consider whose arm would be more stiff/stable.) Less stiffness leads to more movement from application of the same force. If a back is not stiff enough, it will buckle and move under very little force, resulting in compression or stretching of sensitive structures. Pain is the consequence.

Panjabi et al. (1989) proposed the concept of the **neutral zone**—the zone in which movement occurs at the beginning of the range of motion before any effective resistance is offered from either the muscular system or the spinal column. The neutral zone represents the range of motion that lacks effective restraint, either active or passive. It is the vertebral displacement that occurs before resistance is offered. A grossly unstable spinal segment has quite a large neutral zone (figure 1.2). Physiotherapists use this concept when they

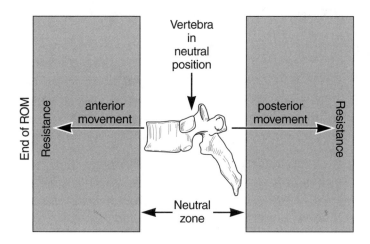

Figure 1.2 The neutral zone.

assess lumbar joint movements by palpation—they note the onset either of motion resistance or of pain as they move the joint. In the case of the lumbar spine in the prone position, movement of this type is usually in a postero-antero (PA) direction. Note that the resistance felt by physiotherapists is mainly passive and does not necessarily represent significant resistance offered by muscle contraction.

The passive stability system (ligaments and bone contour) reduces motion toward the end of the neutral zone. Our strategy, however, is to *reduce the size* of the neutral zone by increasing muscle stability. Exercise that increases muscle stability may reduce motion within the neutral zone before the passive elements even come into play. Note that neutral zone motion is different from the total range of motion—even though stabilizing exercise increases muscle "stiffness," it does not correspondingly reduce the total range of motion. Panjabi (1992) investigated the relationship between total range to neutral zone range by studying the effect of external fixation on the cervical spine in cadavers—and noted that neutral zone motion declined over 70% in association with a decrease of only 40% in total range of motion. In reducing the size of the neutral zone, the back stability program decreases the amount of motion that occurs when minimal forces are imposed on the spine (i.e., those same forces that, when experienced hour after hour, can produce the compression/stretching that lead to back pain). A stable back is not constantly buffeted by minor stresses related to mere sitting, standing, etc., such as those that occur in individuals with unstable spines.

> **KEY POINT:** Instability alters both the quality and quantity of lumbar motion.

Neutral Position of the Lumbar Spine

The neutral position of the lumbar spine is different from the neutral zone. **Lumbar neutral position** refers to an overall movement of the lumbar spine rather than to individual movements between vertebrae. Lumbar neutral position is midway between full flexion and full extension as brought about by posterior and anterior tilting of the pelvis. Teaching patients to identify and maintain the neutral position of their lumbar spines is a key component of each stage of the back stability program, since the neutral position places minimal stress on body tissues. Also, because postural alignment is optimal, the neutral position is generally the most effective position from which trunk muscles can work.

> **KEY POINT:** The neutral position of the lumbar spine is important in all stages of the back stability program because it minimizes stress.

Achieving and Maintaining Spinal Stability

Three interrelated systems maintain spinal stability (figure 1.3). **Inert** tissues (in particular, ligaments) provide passive support; **contractile** tissues give active support; and **neural** control centers coordinate sensory feedback from both systems (Panjabi 1992). Since one or two systems may compensate for reduced stability in another, the active system may sometimes increase its contribution to stability in order to minimize stress on the passive system (Tropp et al. 1993). When the goal of rehabilitation is healing of the spine, appropriate exercise—by enabling the active system to take more of the total load placed on the back—can permit the passive system to repair itself. The net result is decreased pain and increased function. Conversely, continually loading the passive system without proper support from the active system can increase the time to recovery and lead to further tissue damage.

Simply developing muscle strength, however, is insufficient. To provide maximum relief to the passive system, one must augment *both* of the other systems (i.e., the active and neural control systems). Yet many popular strength exercises for the trunk actually increase mobility in this region to dangerously high levels (Norris 1993, 1994a). Rather than improving stability, exercises of this type may reduce it and therefore exacerbate symptoms—especially those associated with inflammation. An example is the bilateral straight-leg-raise movement where both legs are lifted simultaneously from a supine lying position. Although individuals performing this exercise may indeed strengthen their abdominal muscles, they often fail to maintain pelvic alignment. Anterior tilting of the pelvis leads to lumbar facet compression and overstretches the anterior spinal

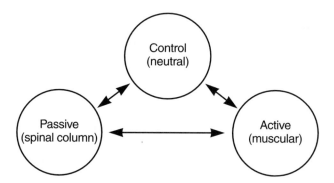

Figure 1.3 The spinal stabilizing system consists of three interrelating subsystems.

Reprinted, by permission, from M.M. Panjabi, 1992, "The stabilisation of the spine. Part 1. Function, dysfunction, adaptation, and enhancement," *Journal of Spinal Disorders* 5(4): 383-389.

tissues. In this case, the anterior longitudinal ligament of the spine may be overstretched, reducing the effect of an important passive stabilizing structure.

Passive Support

Passive support of the lumbar region is provided by the stretching (especially of ligaments) and compression of soft tissues. A compressed ligament is more relaxed and offers less support. In full lumbar extension, for example, as may occur when standing with an anteriorly tilted pelvis, the lumbar facet joints are loaded and compressed. The anterior structures, including the anterior longitudinal ligament, are stretched: stability is provided (passively) through elastic recoil of this ligament and because facet joints of the spine are forcibly closed.

Developing Active Lumbar Stability

Poor postural control can leave the spine vulnerable to injury by placing excessive stress on the body tissues (Kendall et al. 1993). In the lumbar spine, the trunk muscles protect spinal tissues from excessive motion. To do this, however, the muscles surrounding the trunk must be able to co-contract isometrically when appropriate (Richardson et al. 1990). The synergistic interaction between various trunk muscles is complex: some muscles act as prime movers to create the gross movements of the trunk, while others function as stabilizers (fixators) and neutralizers to support the spinal structures and control unwanted movements. Rehabilitation through active lumbar stabilization not only deals with the torque-producing capacity of muscles, as is true of many traditional programs, but also seeks to enable a subject to unconsciously and consistently coordinate an optimal pattern of muscle activity (Jull and Richardson 1994a).

Developing the Neural System

The neural system links the passive and active systems. Upon detecting movement within the neutral zone, the neural system relays information to the active system (muscles) about the position and direction of movement. The muscles' ability to contract and maintain stability (i.e., to increase stiffness and reduce the size of the neutral zone) depends on the speed and accuracy with which the information is relayed. The vital aspects of neural system development are therefore *accuracy of movement* and *speed of reaction*. Thus the stability program emphasizes accuracy of movement early on; speed comes later.

SUMMARY

- Low back pain is a massive challenge to health-care professionals and a major financial drain on Western economies.
- Low back pain produces alterations in behavior patterns that can exacerbate the condition.
- The traditional structural approach to treating back pain must be balanced with restoration of function.
- New approaches to treating back pain emphasize the use of exercise rather than rest.
- Back stability consists of three interrelating control systems: active, passive, and neural.
- Although traditional exercise systems that work the trunk may strengthen muscle, they also may reduce total back stability.
- Enhancing the active and neural systems can partially compensate for decrements in the passive system.
- Enhanced movement accuracy and muscle reaction speed are vital to full rehabilitation of the back.

2

Biomechanics
of the Lumbar Spine

In order to explain how the back is stabilized, I must briefly review some important aspects of spinal anatomy. Chapter 1 describes the passive stability system—the "brakes" provided by inert tissues that will stretch only a certain amount (both individually and as systems of tissues) before they restrict further movement. In this chapter, I describe this passive system for each of the major physiological movements of the lumbar spine and then use the example of lifting to illustrate the importance of stability.

ANATOMY OF THE VERTEBRAL COLUMN

The gross anatomy of the lumbar spine includes vertebral bones, joints, and discs, plus the sacroiliac joints. Although none of these structures moves in isolation, it should prove helpful if I describe them individually.

The Bones and Their Joints

The adult human vertebral column comprises 33 vertebrae. Five vertebrae are fused to form the sacrum and four are fused to form the coccyx. The remaining 24 movable vertebrae are divided among the cervical (7), thoracic (12) and lumbar (5) regions (figure 2.1). Any two neighboring vertebrae make up a **spinal segment** (figure 2.2). To understand how the vertebrae fit together in the spine, one must know the parts of the typical vertebra.

The two vertebrae within a spinal segment are attached (articulated) by both joints and ligaments. There are three joints—the **articulating triad**—consisting of the **disc,** which forms the joint between the bodies of adjacent vertebrae, and the two **facet joints** (also called zygapophyseal or apophyseal joints), where the inferior articular processes on either side of the upper vertebra come together with the superior articular processes on either side of the lower vertebra.

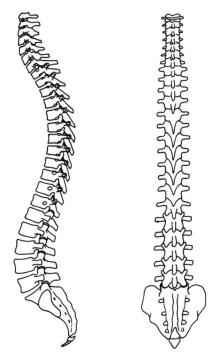

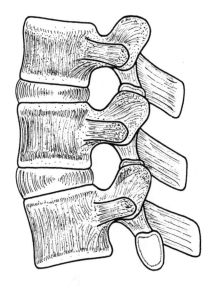

Figure 2.1 The vertebral column.
Reprinted from Watkins 1999.

Figure 2.2 A typical spinal segment.
Reprinted from Watkins 1999.

KEY POINT: A spinal segment comprises two adjacent vertebrae, articulating with each other through the intervertebral disc and two facet joints. The articulations form a triad.

The disk and its associated facet joints are intimately linked both structurally and functionally. Degeneration of the intervertebral disc as a result of injury can lead to degeneration of the neighboring facet joints (Vernon-Roberts 1992); and as we shall see later, the ligamentous support to both structures is continuous.

We can compare the spinal segment to a simple leverage system (Kapandji 1974), with the facet joints forming a fulcrum. The posterior tissues (ligamentous and muscular) and the anteriorly placed disc resist both compressive and tensile forces. The ligaments themselves may be categorized into three interrelating functional groups as shown in table 2.1.

Ligaments

The neural arch ligaments consist mainly of the ligamentum flavum and the interspinous ligament, with the supraspinous and intertransverse

Table 2.1 Ligaments of the Spinal Segment

Neural arch	Capsular	Ventral
▪ Ligamentum flavum ▪ Interspinous ligament ▪ Supraspinous ligament ▪ Intertransverse ligament	▪ Facet joint capsule (reinforced by the ligamentum flavum)	▪ Anterior longitudinal ligament ▪ Posterior longitudinal ligament

Adapted, by permission, from F.H. Willard, 1997, The muscular, ligamentous and neural structure of the low back and its relation to back pain. In *Movement stability and low back pain*, edited by A. Vleeming, V. Mooney, T. Dorman, C. Snijders, and R. Stoeckart (Edinburgh: Churchill Livingstone).

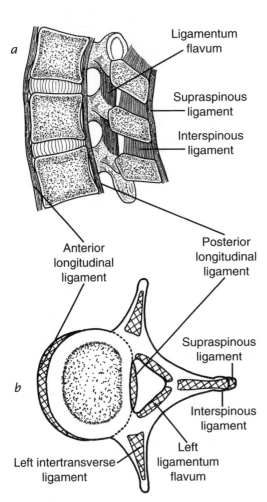

Ligamentum flavum

Supraspinous ligament

Interspinous ligament

Anterior longitudinal ligament

Posterior longitudinal ligament

Supraspinous ligament

Interspinous ligament

Left intertransverse ligament

Left ligamentum flavum

Figure 2.3 Ligaments of the spinal segment *(a)* side view, *(b)* superior view.

ligaments providing additional support (figure 2.3 a and b). Although these four ligaments are traditionally described as separate structures, they are actually merged at their edges and act functionally as a single unit. This is an extremely important point, as it bears significantly on the question of how one stabilizes the back. On dissection, when the bony components of the neural arch are removed, the neural arch ligaments can be seen to maintain their continuity (Willard 1997). The lateral fibers of the ligamentum flavum are continuous with the facet joint capsule (Yong-Hing et al. 1976) and form the rear wall of the spinal canal. The anterior border of the interspinous ligament is a continuation of the ligamentum flavum, while the posterior border of this ligament is thickened into the supraspinous ligament. The supraspinous ligament merges with the thoracolumbar fascia (TLF) (figure 2.4), which in turn connects

Terms You Should Know

articulate to join or connect loosely to allow motion between the connection, such as a joint

caudal any tail-like structure

contralateral fibers fibers originating in or affecting the opposite side of the body

distraction force a force that separates a joint surface without injury or dislocation

extension a movement that straightens a limb to a parallel or near-parallel position

fascia a sheet of fibrous tissue under the skin that encloses muscles as well as separates and supports them; connects the skin with the tissue beneath it

flexion bending or being bent; opposite of extension

innominate bone the hip bone composed of the ilium, ischium, and pubis; forms the pelvis

investing fascia fascia that surrounds rather than connects or separates

ischemic deficiency of blood to a body part due to an obstruction in or a narrowing of the blood vessels

lamina of vertebral arch the posterior portion of the arch that provides a base for the spine

lateral flexion bending or being bent to the side

lordosis inward curvature of the cervical and lumbar spines

occiput the back part of the head

vertebral pedicle the bony process that extends posteriorly from the body of a vertebra; one of the paired parts of the vertebral arch that connect the lamina to the vertebral body

pelvic inlet the upper opening of the pelvis

pelvic outlet the lower opening of the pelvis

periosteum a thick, fibrous membrane covering all the bones of the body except at the joints

prolapse downward displacement

sagittal rotation turning from the front to the back

sagittal plane a vertical plane through the body that divides it into the left and right side

Schmorls node an irregular or hemispherical bone defect in the body of a vertebra, which a spinal disk herniates into

trabecula fibrous cord of connective tissue that extends into an organ's wall to serve as support

ventral front side of the body

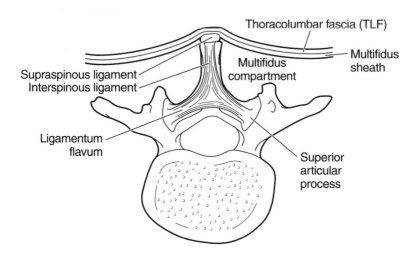

Figure 2.4 Interspinous-supraspinous-thoracolumbar (IST) ligamentous complex. The IST complex supports the lumbar spine by anchoring the thoracolumbar fascia and multifidus sheath to the facet joint capsules

with the deep abdominal muscles (see page 57). The force generated by the deep abdominal muscles therefore can be transmitted through the TLF, via the supraspinous ligament, directly into the ligamentum flavum—preventing this ligament from buckling towards the spinal cord. This is one way the deep abdominals assist in spinal stabilization.

Note that it is not only abdominal muscles that affect the spine. The interspinous ligament merges with the supraspinous ligament and then into the TLF, forming the interspinous-supraspinous-thoracolumbar (IST) ligamentous complex (Willard 1997). The IST complex attaches the fascia of the back to the lumbar spine. The importance of this system is that tension developed *in the extremities* is transmitted to the vertebral column, making the seemingly distant limb musculature essential to the rehabilitation of spinal function. The intertransverse ligament, although small, becomes more important caudally as it expands into the iliolumbar ligament, the importance of which I will discuss later.

> **KEY POINT:** Force from the extremity muscles is transmitted to the spine via ligaments and fasciae, which ultimately attach to the vertebrae themselves. The deep abdominal muscles have the greatest capacity to stabilize the spine.

The capsule of the facet joint is reinforced posteriorly by the multifidus muscle and anteriorly by the ligamentum flavum. It is surrounded by fascia which is itself continuous with that covering the ligamentum flavum and the investing fascia of the vertebral body. The facet joint capsule therefore can be seen as a "bridge" of connective tissue between the ligaments of the neural arch and those of the vertebral body (Willard 1997) (figure 2.5).

The anterior longitudinal ligament (ALL) and posterior longitudinal ligament (PLL) lie ventrally within the spinal segment. The ALL is the stronger of the two and extends from the occiput to the sacrum where it merges with the sacroiliac joint capsule. The ALL has two sets of fibers (Bogduk and Twomey 1991). The superficial fibers span several vertebral segments, while the deep fibers attach loosely to the annulus of the spinal disc (figure 2.6). The PLL exists in the cervical spine as the tectorial membrane and extends caudally to the periosteum of the sacrum. It expands as it passes the intervertebral discs and narrows around the vertebral body. Because it is considerably weaker than the ALL, the main ligamentous restriction to flexion is not from the PLL but from the ligamentum flavum and the facet joint capsule into which it merges. The ligamentum flavum and facet joint capsules combine to offer 52% of the resistance to flexion in the lumbar spine (Bogduk and Twomey 1991). The structural pairing of the PLL and the ligamentum flavum is functionally obvious as well. Load-deformation (stress-strain) curves plotted for the two ligaments are similar (Panjabi and White 1990), suggesting in this case that the two ligaments may have a similar purpose.

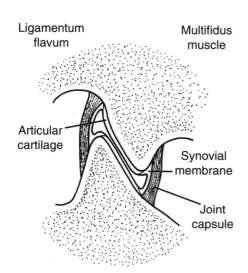

Figure 2.5 Facet joint capsule.

Reprinted from Watkins 1999.

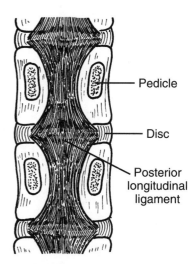

Figure 2.6 Vertical section through pedicles in lumbar region: posterior aspect of vertebral bodies showing attachment of posterior longitudinal ligament to spinal discs.

Reprinted from Watkins 1999.

The longitudinal ligaments are viscoelastic, meaning that they stiffen when loaded rapidly. They do not store all the energy used to stretch them because they lose some as heat, a feature known as *hysteresis*. When loaded repeatedly, these ligaments become even stiffer, and the hysteresis is less marked, making them more prone to fatigue failure (Hukins 1987). The supraspinous and interspinous ligaments are farther from the flexion axis and therefore need to stretch more than the posterior longitudinal ligament when they resist flexion.

With age, all ligaments gradually lose their ability to absorb energy (Tkaczuk 1968). The stiffest ligament in the spine is the posterior longitudinal ligament; the most flexible is the supraspinous (Panjabi et al. 1987). The ligamentum flavum in the lumbar spine is "pretensioned" (possesses tension at rest) when the spine is in its neutral position, a situation that compresses the spinal disc. This ligament has the highest percentage of elastic fibers of any tissue in the body (Nachemson and Evans 1968) and contains nearly twice as much elastin as collagen. The anterior longitudinal ligament and joint capsules are among the strongest ligamentous tissues in the body, while the interspinous and posterior longitudinal ligaments are the weakest (Panjabi et al. 1987).

KEY POINT: The ligamentum flavum is the most elastic ligament in the body and the main ligament limiting flexion. It forms the anterior portion of the facet joint capsule.

Spinal Discs

There are 24 intervertebral discs lying between successive vertebrae, making the spine an alternatively rigid then elastic column. The amount of flexibility in a particular spinal segment is determined by the size and shape of the disc and by the resistance to motion of the soft tissue that supports the spinal joints. The discs increase in size as they descend the column, the lumbar discs having an average thickness of 10 mm, twice that of the cervical discs. The disc shapes are accommodated to the curvatures of the spine and to the shapes of the vertebrae. The greater anterior widths of the discs in the cervical and lumbar regions reflect the curvatures of these areas. Each disc comprises three closely related components—the annulus fibrosis, nucleus pulposus, and cartilage end plates (figure 2.7).

The annulus comprises layers of fibrous tissue arranged in concentric bands—about 20—like those in an onion. The fibers within each band are parallel, with the various bands angled at 45° to each other. The bands are more closely packed anteriorly and posteriorly than they are laterally, and those innermost are the thinnest. Fiber orientation, although partially determined at birth, is influenced by torsional stresses in the adult (Palastanga

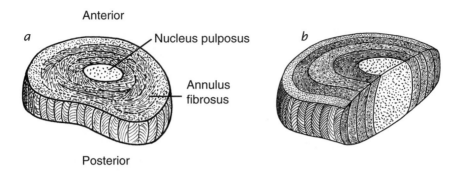

Figure 2.7 *(a)* Concentric bands of annular fibers. *(b)* Horizontal section through a disc.

Reprinted, by permission, from J. Watkins, 1999, *Structure and function of the musculoskeletal system* (Champaign, IL: Human Kinetics), 142.

et al. 1994). The posterolateral regions have a more irregular makeup—possibly one reason why they become weaker with aging and more predisposed to injury.

KEY POINT: The spinal discs have fewer concentric bands posterolaterally than in other regions, and these are irregular—making this region of the disc more susceptible to injury.

The annular fibers pass over the edge of the cartilage end plate of the disc and are anchored to the bony rim of the vertebra and to its periosteum and body. The attaching fibers are actually interwoven with the fibers of the bony trabeculae of the vertebral body. The outer layer of fibers blend with the posterior longitudinal ligament; some authors claim that the anterior longitudinal ligament has no such attachment (Vernon-Roberts 1987).

Resting on the surface of the vertebra, the hyaline cartilage end plate is approximately 1 mm thick at its outer edge and becomes thinner toward its center. The central portion of the end plate acts as a semipermeable membrane to facilitate fluid exchange into and out of the disc; it also protects the vertebral body from excessive pressure. In early life, canals from the vertebral body penetrate the end plate, but these disappear after the age of 20 to 30. The end plate then starts to ossify and become more brittle, while the central portion thins and, in some cases, is completely destroyed.

The nucleus pulposus is a soft hydrophilic (water-attracting) substance taking up about 25% of the total disc area. It is continuous with the annulus, but the nuclear fibers are far less dense than those of the annulus. Mucopolysaccharides called *proteoglycans* fill the spaces between the collagen fibers of the nucleus, giving the nucleus its water-retaining capacity and making it mechanically plastic. Metabolically very active, the area between the nucleus and annulus is sensitive both to physical force and to chemical/hormonal influence (Palastanga et al. 1994). Although the collagen volume of the nucleus remains unchanged, the proteoglycan content decreases with age—leading to a net reduction in water content. In early life, the water content may be as high as 80-90%, but this decreases to about 70% by middle age.

The lumbar discs are the largest avascular structures in the body. The nucleus obtains fluids by passive diffusion from the margins of the vertebral body and across the cartilage end plate—particularly across the center of the end plate, which is more permeable than the periphery. Intense anaerobic activity within the nucleus (Holm et al. 1981) can lead to lactate buildup and low oxygen concentration, placing the nuclear cells at risk. Inadequate ATP levels may lead to cell death. Some researchers hypothesize that regular exercise involving movement of the spine may improve the nutrition of the disc—and over the years might not only improve the general health of discs, but even slow the loss of height due to water loss from discs.

KEY POINT: The lumbar spinal discs are avascular and depend on fluid exchange by passive diffusion. Regular movement/activity is vital to this process.

Facet Joints

The facet joints are synovial joints (cushioned by synovia, a viscous fluid) between the inferior articular process of one vertebra and the superior articular process of its neighbor. As with other typical synovial joints, they have articular cartilage, a synovial membrane to contain the fluid, and a joint capsule; but they also have a number of unique features (Bogduk and Twomey 1991).

The facet joint capsule holds about 2 ml of synovial fluid. Its anterior wall is formed by the ligamentum flavum; posteriorly, the capsule is reinforced by the deep fibers of the multifidus muscle. At its superior and inferior poles, the joint leaves a small gap, creating the subscapular pockets. These are filled with fat, contained within the synovial membrane. Within the subscapular pocket lies a small foramen for passage of the fat in and out of the joint as the spine moves.

Within the capsule, there are three structures of interest. The first is the connective tissue rim, a thickened wedge-shaped area that makes up for the curved shape of the articular cartilage in much the same way as the menisci of the knee do. The second structure is an adipose tissue pad, a 2-mm fold of synovium filled with fat and blood vessels. The third structure is the fibroadipose meniscoid, a 5-mm leaf-like fold that projects from the inner surfaces of the superior and inferior capsules. The last two structures have a protective function. Flexion leaves some of the articular facets' cartilage exposed—both the adipose tissue pad and the fibro-adipose meniscus cover the exposed regions (Bogduk and Engel 1984).

With aging, cartilage of the facet joint can split parallel to the joint surface, pulling a portion of joint capsule with it. The split cartilage, with its attached piece of capsule, forms a false intra-articular meniscoid (Taylor and Twomey 1986). Flexion normally draws the fibro-adipose meniscus out from the joint, and it moves back in with extension. If the meniscus fails to move back, it will buckle and remain under the capsule, causing pain (Bogduk and Jull 1985). A mobilization or manipulation that combines flexion and rotation may relieve pain by allowing the meniscoid to move back into its original position.

The Sacroiliac Joint

As with the lumbar spine, the sacroiliac joint (SIJ)—the rather large surface where the sacrum (the five fused bottom vertebrae of the spine) fits into the pelvis (figure 2.8)—is stabilized by several ligaments that connect to muscles within the region. The iliolumbar ligament attaches to the transverse process of L5, and in some subjects to those of L4 as well (Willard 1997), and passes anteromedially to the iliac crest and the surface of the

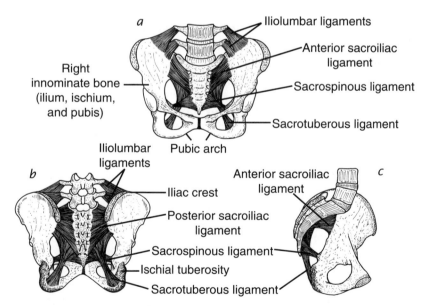

Figure 2.8 The sacroiliac joint and its supporting ligaments: *(a)* anterior aspect; *(b)* posterior aspect; and *(c)* left aspect of medial section through the pelvis.

Reprinted, by permission, from J. Watkins, 1999, *Structure and function of the musculoskeletal system* (Champaign, IL: Human Kinetics), 1972.

ilium. The iliolumbar ligament resists movement between the sacrum and lumbar spine, particularly that of lateral flexion. When the ligament is cut, movement of the lumbar spine (L5) on the sacrum increases significantly—lateral flexion by nearly 30%; and flexion, extension, and rotation by 18-23% (Yamamoto et al. 1990). The superior aspect of the SIJ capsule is an extension of the iliolumbar ligament, while the anterior portion of the capsule merges into the sacrotuberous ligament.

The sacrotuberous ligament has a triangular shape extending between the posterior iliac spines, SIJ capsule, and coccyx (figure 2.8). Importantly, the tendon of biceps femoris (the large muscle at the back of the upper leg) extends over the ischial tuberosity to attach to the sacrotuberous ligament (Vleeming et al. 1989); the ligament also attaches into some of the deepest fibers of the multifidus muscle (the multifidus runs vertically down the entire length of the back, on either side of the spine) (Willard 1997). Movement at the sacroiliac joint is described as nutation and counternutation (table 2.2). The sacrotuberous ligament resists nutation of the sacrum, while the long dorsal sacroiliac ligament resists counternutation.

Even though it is difficult to discern this from observing most anatomical diagrams, the sacrum is not fused with the pelvis—so when I speak of movement of the sacrum, I mean motion *within* the pelvis as opposed to motion *of* the pelvis, where the entire structure is moving on the hip. Greater movement ranges have been reported in nonweightbearing than weightbearing movements. Nonweightbearing movements have exhibited as much as 12° innominate rotation during flexion, together with 8 mm translation during extension (Lavignolle et al. 1983); weightbearing movements were reduced to 2.5° rotation and 1.6 mm maximal transla-

Table 2.2 Movement of the Sacroiliac Joint (SIJ)

Nutation	Counternutation
■ Anterior tilting of sacrum	■ Posterior tilting of sacrum
■ Sacral base moves down and forward, apex moves up	■ Sacral base moves up and back, apex moves down
■ Size of pelvic outlet increased, pelvic inlet decreased	■ Pelvic inlet increased, outlet reduced
■ Occurs in standing	■ Occurs in nonweightbearing position such as lying
■ Increased as lumbar lordosis increased	■ Increased as lumbar lordosis decreased (flatback posture)
■ Iliac bones pulled together, SIJ impacted	■ Iliac bones move apart, SIJ distracted
■ Superior aspect of pubis compressed	■ Inferior aspect of pubis compressed

tion (Sturesson et al. 1989). In a study of healthy individuals aged 20-50 years, Jacob and Kissling (1995) found average rotational motion at the SIJ to be 2°, whereas symptomatic patients averaged 6°.

Nutation of the SIJ is an anterior tilting of the sacrum on the fixed innominate bones. The sacral base moves down and forward, while the sacral apex moves up, increasing the pelvic outlet. Nutation occurs in standing and increases as lordosis deepens. By pulling the iliac bones together, nutation compresses the SIJ as well as the superior portion of the pubic symphasis. **Counternutation** is the opposite movement, with the sacral base moving up and back and the apex moving downward. This movement occurs in nonweightbearing situations, such as lying prone, and increases as the lordosis is reduced and the low back is flattened. During counternutation, the iliac bones move apart, the pelvic inlet increases, and the pelvic outlet reduces (Kesson and Atkins 1998).

A variety of movements occur about the SIJ during trunk actions (Lee 1994). During forward bending of the trunk, the pelvis tilts anteriorly and the sacrum moves into extension (coccyx moving backward; i.e., nutation around an oblique axis), causing the iliac crests and posterior superior iliac spines (PSIS) to approximate (i.e., press toward each other) and the ischial tuberosities and the anterior superior iliac spines (ASIS) to separate. During side bending, the trunk laterally flexes and the pelvis shifts to the opposite direction to maintain balance. With left lateral flexion and right pelvic shift, the right innominate bone rotates posteriorly, and the left innominate rotates anteriorly. The sacrum rotates to the right. During trunk rotation, the pelvis rotates in the same direction; therefore, with left trunk rotation, the right innominate anteriorly rotates and the left posteriorly rotates. The sacrum is driven into left rotation.

AXIAL COMPRESSION

Vertical loading of the lumbar spine (axial compression) occurs during upright (standing or sitting) postures, exacerbating certain forms of back pain. Knowledge of loading can help us to design safer exercise programs for the back pain sufferer.

Compression of the Vertebral Bodies

Within the vertebra itself, compressive force is transmitted by both the cancellous (spongy) bone of the vertebral body and its cortical bone shell. Until about the age of 40, the cancellous bone contributes about 25-55% of the vertebra's strength. As aging-related decreases in bone density lead to a decline in the proportion of cancellous bone, the cortical bone shell carries a greater proportion of load (Rockoff et al. 1969). As the vertebral body is compressed, a net flow of blood out of it (Crock and Yoshizawa

1976) reduces bone volume and dissipates energy (Roaf 1960). Blood returns slowly as the force is reduced—leaving a latent period after the initial compression and diminishing the shock-absorbing properties of the bone. Exercises that involve prolonged periods of repeated shock to the spine (e.g., jumping on a hard surface) are therefore more likely to damage vertebrae than those that load the spine for short periods and allow recovery of the vertebral blood flow before repeating a movement.

KEY POINT: Blood flows out of the vertebral body with loading, decreasing its shock-absorbing properties. Exercises that repeatedly load the spine without allowing recovery can therefore lead to accumulated stress.

Compression of Intervertebral Discs

During standing, 12-25% of axial compression forces are transmitted between adjacent vertebrae by the facet joints (see discussion on page 28); the intervertebral disc absorbs the rest of the force (Miller et al. 1983). The annulus fibrosis of a healthy disc resists buckling; even if a disc's nucleus pulposus has been removed, its annulus alone can exhibit a loadbearing capacity similar to that of the fully intact disc *for a brief period* (Markolf and Morris 1974). When exposed to prolonged loading however, the collagen lamellae of the annulus eventually buckle (see figure 2.7).

Throughout the waking day, discal loading diminishes a person's height until the forces inside the disc equal the load forces (Twomey and Taylor 1994). By reducing axial loading, lying down permits restoration of the former spinal length. Lying in a flexed position speeds the regain of lost height as the lumbar discs are distracted (unloaded) during flexion (Tyrrell et al. 1985). Application of an axial load compresses the fluid nucleus of the disc, causing it to expand laterally. This lateral expansion stretches the annular fibers, preventing them from buckling. The degree of discal compression depends on the weight imposed and the rate of loading. A 100-kg axial load can compress a disc by 1.4 mm and cause a lateral expansion of 0.75 mm (Hirsch and Nachemson 1954). The stretch in the annular fibers stores energy, which is released when the compression stress is removed. The stored energy gives the disc a certain springiness, which helps to offset any deformation that occurred in the nucleus. A force applied rapidly is not lessened by this mechanism, but its rate of application is slowed, giving the spinal tissues time to adapt.

Deformation of the disc occurs more rapidly at the onset of axial load application, the majority of its deformation occurring within 10 minutes of onset. After this time, deformation continues but slows to a rate of about 1 mm per hour (Markolf and Morris 1974), leading to loss of height throughout the day. Under constant loading the discs exhibit "creep" (i.e., they continue to deform even though the load is not increasing). Because compression causes a rise in fluid pressure, fluid is actually lost from both the nucleus and the annulus. About 10% of the water within the disc can be squeezed out by this method (Kraemer et al. 1985), the exact amount dependent on the size and duration of the applied force. When the compressive force is reduced, the fluid is absorbed back through pores in the cartilage end plates of the vertebra. Exercises that axially load the spine reduce a person's height through discal compression—squat exercises in weight training, for example, can create compression loads in the L3-L4 segment of 6-10 times bodyweight (Cappozzo et al. 1985). Researchers have observed average height losses of 5.4 mm over a 25-minute period of general weight training, and 3.25 mm after a 6-km run (Leatt et al. 1986) (figure 2.9). Static axial loading of the spine with a 40-kg barbell over a 20-minute period can reduce a subject's height by as much as 11.2 mm (Tyrrell et al. 1985). Clearly, exercises that involve this degree of spinal loading are unsuitable for individuals with discal pathology.

The vertebral end plates of the discs are compressed centrally and are able to undergo less deformation than either the annulus or the cancellous bone. The end plates are therefore likely to fail (fracture) under high compression (Norkin and Levangie 1992). Discs subjected to very high compressive loads can show permanent deformation without herniation (Farfan et al. 1976; Markolf and Morris 1974). However, such compression forces may lead to **Schmorls node** formation (Bernhardt et al. 1992): the disc end plate (which joins the disc to the vertebral body) ruptures, and nuclear material from the disc passes through to the vertebral body itself. Bending and torsional stresses on the spine, when combined with compression, are more damaging than compression alone, and degenerated discs are particularly at risk. Average failure torques for normal discs are

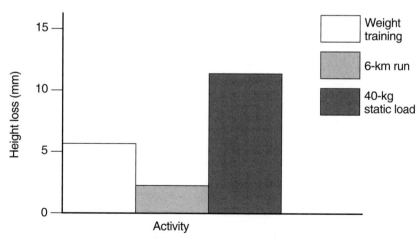

Figure 2.9 Discal compression and height loss during exercise.

25% higher than for degenerative discs (Farfan et al. 1976). Degenerative discs also demonstrate poorer viscoelastic properties and therefore a reduced ability to attenuate shock.

The proteoglycan of the disc's nucleus makes it hydrophilic, and its ability to transmit load relies on high water content; yet proteoglycan content declines from about 65% in early life to about 30% by middle age (Bogduk and Twomey 1987). When the proteoglycan content of the disc is high (up to age 30 in most subjects), the nucleus pulposus is gelatinous, producing a uniform fluid pressure. After this age, the lower water content of the disc leaves the nucleus unable to build as much fluid pressure. Less central pressure is produced, and the load is distributed more peripherally, eventually causing the annular fibers to become fibrillated and to crack (Hirsch and Schajowicz 1952). The net result is that a disc's reaction to compressive stress declines with age (figure 2.10).

The age-related changes in discs cause greater susceptibility to injury. This fact—combined with a general reduction in fitness and changes in trunk movement patterns related to activities of daily living—greatly increases the risk of injury in older individuals. Encourage previously inactive persons over the age of 40 to engage in trunk exercises, under the supervision of a physiotherapist, before attending fitness classes.

Compression of Facet Joints

The orientations of facet joints differ among various regions of the spine, thereby altering the available motion. In the mid- and lower cervical spine, for example, rotation and lateral flexion are limited but flexion and extension are possible. In the thoracic spine, flexion and extension are limited but lateral flexion and rotation are free. At the thoracolumbar junction (T12-L1), rotation is the only movement that is limited; in the lumbar spine, both rotation and lateral flexion are limited.

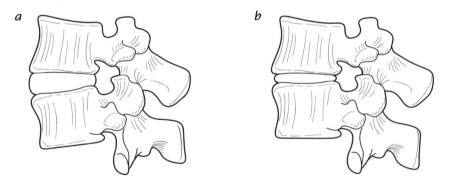

Figure 2.10 Age-related changes in lumbar discs. *(a)* Maximal disc height and end plate length of youth. *(b)* Reduced measurements through aging.

The superior/inferior alignment of the facet joints in the lumbar spine means that, during axial loading in the neutral position, the joint surfaces slide past each other. Note, however, that anywhere between T9 and T12, the orientation of the facet joints may change from those characteristic of the thoracic spine to those of the lumbar spine. Therefore, the level at which particular movements will occur can vary considerably among subjects. During lumbar movements, displacement of the facet joint surfaces causes them to impact, or press together. Because the sacrum is inclined and the body and disc of L5 are wedge shaped, during axial loading L5 is subjected to a shearing force. This force is resisted by the more anterior orientation of the L5 inferior articular processes. As the lordosis increases, moreover, the anterior longitudinal ligament and the anterior portion of the annulus fibrosis are stretched, providing tension to resist the bending force. Additional stabilization is provided for the L5 vertebra by the iliolumbar ligament, attached to the L5 transverse process. This ligament, together with the facet joint capsules, stretches to resist the distraction force.

Once the axial compression force stops, release of the stored elastic energy in the spinal ligaments re-establishes the neutral lordosis. With compression of the lordotic lumbar spine, or in cases where gross disc narrowing has occurred, the inferior articular processes may impact on the lamina of the vertebra below (see figure 2.11). In this case, the lower joints (L3/4, L4/5, L5/S1) may bear as much as 19% of the compression force, while the upper joints (L1/2, L2/3) bear only 11% (Adams et al. 1980).

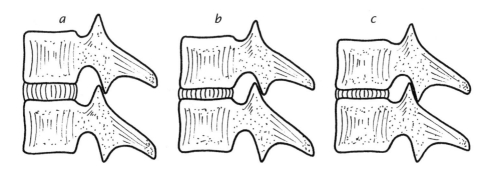

Figure 2.11 Results of compression on discs and facet joints. *(a)* Normal disc thickness and alignment of superior and inferior articular processes. *(b)* Reduced disc thickness resulting in increased compression load on facet joint. *(c)* Extra-articular impingement of facet joint.

Reprinted, by permission, from J. Watkins, 1999, *Structure and function of the musculoskeletal system* (Champaign, IL: Human Kinetics), 146.

MOVEMENTS OF THE LUMBAR SPINE AND PELVIS

Much of the material for this section comes from Norris (1995a) and Norris (1998), to which I refer you for further reading.

Flexion and Extension

Both disc height and the horizontal length of the vertebral end plate affect the range of motion attainable during sagittal plane movement of the lumbar spine. Greatest range of motion occurs with a combination of maximum disc height and maximum end plate length (figure 2.10). Since this alignment most often occurs in young females, it is they who possess the greatest ranges of motion at the lumbar spine. With aging, disc height and end plate length become more similar between the sexes, equalizing the available range of motion for males and females in old age (Twomey and Taylor 1994).

During flexion movements, the anterior annulus of a lumbar disc is compressed, whereas the posterior fibers are stretched. Similarly, the nucleus pulposus of the disc is compressed anteriorly, whereas pressure is relieved over its posterior surface. Since the total volume of the disc remains unchanged, however, its pressure should not increase. The increases in pressure seen with posture changes are due not to the bending motion of the bones within the vertebral joint itself but to the soft tissue tension created to control the bending. If the pressure at the L3 disc for a 70-kg standing subject is said to be 100%, supine lying reduces the pressure to 25%. The pressure variations increase dramatically as soon as the lumbar spine is flexed and tissue tension increases (figure 2.12). The sitting posture increases intradiscal pressure to 140%, whereas sitting and leaning for-

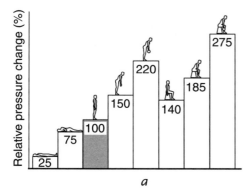

a

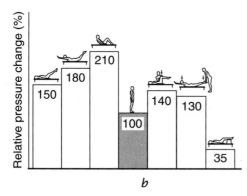

b

Figure 2.12 Pressure changes in the third lumbar disc: *(a)* in different positions; *(b)* in different muscle-strengthening exercises.

From Norris 1998.

ward with a 10-kg weight in each hand increases pressure to 275% (Nachemson 1992). The selection of an appropriate starting position for trunk exercises is therefore of great importance. Spinal exercise from a slumped sitting posture, for example, places considerably more stress on spinal discs than the same movement beginning from crook lying (lying on the back with the knees and hips flexed, feet flat on the floor).

The posterior annulus stretches during flexion, whereas the nucleus is compressed onto the posterior wall. Since the posterior portion of the annulus is the thinnest part, the combination of stretch and pressure to this area may result in discal bulging or herniation. Because layers of annular fibers alternate in direction, rotation movements stretch only half of the fibers at any given time. The disc is more easily injured during a *combination* of rotation and flexion, which stretches all the fibers at the same time.

As the lumbar spine flexes, the lordosis flattens and then reverses at its upper levels. Reversal of lordosis does not occur at L5-S1 (Pearcy et al. 1984). Flexion of the lumbar spine involves a combination of anterior sagittal rotation and anterior translation. As sagittal rotation occurs, the articular facets move apart, permitting the translation movement to occur. Translation is limited by impaction of the inferior facet of one vertebra on the superior facet of the vertebra below. As flexion increases, or if the spine is angled forward on the hip, the surface (i.e., the top) of the vertebral body faces more vertically, increasing the shearing force due to gravity. The forces involved in facet impaction therefore increase to limit translation of the vertebra and stabilize the lumbar spine. Because the facet joint has a curved articular facet, the load is not concentrated evenly across the whole surface but is focused on the anteromedial portion of the facets (figure 2.13).

The sagittal rotation movement of the facet joint causes the joint to open and is therefore limited by the stretch of the joint capsule. The posteriorly placed spinal ligaments are also tightened. Adams et al. (1980) used mathematical modeling to analyze the forces that limit sagittal rotation within the lumbar spine. They found that the disc contributes 29% of the limit to movement, the supraspinous and interspinous ligaments 19%, and the facet joint capsules 39%. In one experiment, the researchers cut (and thereby "released") various posterior tissues in cadavers in order to measure the effects of those tissues on flexion range. Range of motion increased about 4° when the posterior ligaments were released and 9° when the capsule was released. Releasing the pedicles increased the flexion range by 24° in young (14-22 years) subjects. Cutting all the posterior elements increased the flexion range by 100% in the young subjects but by only 60% in the elderly (61-78 years) subjects.

During sustained flexion, tissue overstretch results in creep—gradually increasing the range of motion as tissues elongate over time. With aging, the amount of creep is greater, but recovery takes longer (Twomey and

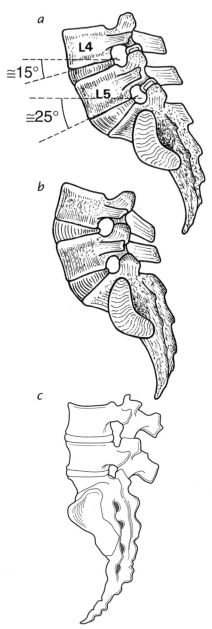

Figure 2.13 The lower lumbar spine and sacrum in *(a)* standing, *(b)* extension, and *(c)* flexion.

Reprinted, by permission, from J. Watkins, 1999, *Structure and function of the musculoskeletal system* (Champaign, IL: Human Kinetics), 147.

Taylor 1994). Occupations that involve prolonged flexion with little recovery (e.g., bricklaying or sitting with poor posture) provide little chance for the overstretched tissue to recover, leading to chronic adaptation of both soft tissue and bone. Such individuals suffer from a high incidence of chronic postural back pain with many acute episodes (Twomey et al. 1988).

KEY POINT: Sustained flexion results in creep of the lumbar tissues (i.e., a gradual increase in range of motion over time). Prolonged flexion with inadequate tissue recovery can lead to chronic adaptation and consequent pain.

During extension, anterior structures are under tension, whereas posterior structures are first taken off stretch and then compressed (depending on the range of motion). Extension movements subject the vertebral bodies to posterior sagittal rotation. The inferior articular processes move downward, causing them to impact against the lamina of the vertebra below. Once the bony block has occurred, if further load is applied, the upper vertebra will axially rotate by pivoting on the impacted inferior articular process. The inferior articular process will move backward, overstretching and possibly damaging the joint capsule (Yang and King 1984). Repeated movements of this type eventually can lead to erosion of the laminal periosteum (Oliver and Middleditch 1991). At the site of impaction, the joint capsule may catch between the opposing bones, creating another source of pain (Adams and Hutton 1983). Since structural abnormalities can alter a vertebra's axis of rotation, considerable variation exists among subjects (Klein and Hukins 1983).

Rotation and Lateral Flexion

During rotation, torsional stiffness is provided by the outer layers of the annulus, by the orientation of the facet joints, and by the cortical bone shell of the vertebral bodies themselves. Moreover, the annular fibers of the disc are stretched as their orientation permits—since alternating layers of fibers are angled obliquely to each other, some fibers will be stretched while others relax. A maximum range of 3° of rotation can occur before the annular fibers will be microscopically damaged and a maximum of 12° before tissue failure (Bogduk and Twomey 1987). The spinous processes separate during rotation, stretching the supraspinous and interspinous ligaments. **Impaction** occurs between the opposing articular facets on one side, causing the articular cartilage to compress by 0.5 mm for each 1° of rotation and providing a substantial buffer mechanism (Bogduk and Twomey 1987). If rotation continues beyond this point, the vertebra pivots around the impacted facet joint, causing posterior and lateral movement. The combination of movements and forces stress the impacted facet joint by compression, the spinal disc by torsion and shear, and the capsule of the opposite facet joint by traction. The disc provides only 35% of the total resistance (Farfan et al. 1976).

When the lumbar spine is laterally flexed, the annular fibers toward the concavity of the curve are compressed and begin to bulge, while those on the convexity of the curve are stretched. The contralateral fibers of the outer annulus and the contralateral intertransverse ligaments help to resist extremes of motion (Norkin and Levangie 1992). Lateral flexion and rotation occur as **coupled movements.** In the neutral position, rotation of the upper four lumbar segments is accompanied by lateral flexion to the opposite side; rotation of the L5-S1 joint, however, occurs with lateral flexion to the same side. The nature of the coupling varies with the degree of flexion and extension. In the neutral position, rotation and lateral flexion occur to the *opposite* side, called "type I movement" (i.e., right rotation is coupled with left lateral flexion). But when the lumbar spine is in flexion or extension, rotation and lateral flexion occur in the *same* direction, called "type II movement" (i.e., right rotation is coupled with right lateral flexion). In the concavity of lateral flexion, the inferior facet of the upper vertebra slides downward on the superior facet of the vertebra below, reducing the area of the intervertebral foramen on that side. On the convexity of the laterally flexed spine, the inferior facet slides upwards on the superior facet of the vertebra below, increasing the diameter of the intervertebral foramen.

Lumbar-Pelvic Rhythm

When people bend forward as though to touch their toes, the movement comes from both the pelvis and the lumbar spine. The pelvis anteriorly tilts on the femur, while the lumbar spine flexes on the pelvis. The combined movement of both lumbar and pelvic motion is called "lumbar-pelvic rhythm." With the lumbar spine held immobile and the knees locked, the pelvis can tilt only to roughly 90° hip flexion (hamstring tightness limits further movement). To touch the floor, one must also flex the lumbar spine. Similarly, with the pelvis held immobile, lumbar flexion is limited to about 30-40°, with most movement occurring at the lower lumbar segments. Therefore, to achieve full forward bending, one must move both body segments. When flexing to midrange levels during daily living, individuals can significantly reduce their lumbar flexion by using anterior pelvic tilt. Reduced ability to anteriorly tilt the pelvis increases the need to flex the lumbar spine, opening the possibility of postural pain through repetitive loading of the lumbar tissues.

When a person bends forward from a standing position, the pelvis and lumbar spine rotate in the same direction. Lumbar flexion accompanies anterior tilt of the pelvis (figure 2.14a). In the upright posture, the feet and shoulders are static, and the pelvis and lumbar spine move in opposite directions (figure 2.14b)—lumbar extension compensates for an anteriorly tilted pelvis in order to maintain the head and shoulders in an upright orientation. Table 2.3 describes the relationship between various pelvic movements and the corresponding hip joint action.

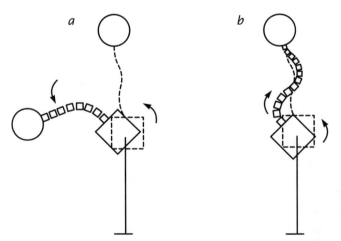

Figure 2.14 (a) Lumbar-pelvic rhythm in open chain formation occurs in the same direction. Anterior pelvic tilt accompanies lumbar flexion. (b) Lumbar-pelvic rhythm in closed kinetic chain formation occurs in opposite directions. Anterior pelvic tilt is compensated by lumbar extension.

From Norris 1998.

Table 2.3   Relationship of Pelvis, Hip Joint, and Lumbar Spine During Right Lower-Extremity Weightbearing and Upright Posture

Pelvic motion	Accompanying hip joint motion	Compensatory lumbar motion
Anterior pelvic tilt	Hip flexion	Lumbar extension
Posterior pelvic tilt	Hip extension	Lumbar flexion
Lateral pelvic tilt (pelvic drop)	Right hip adduction	Right lateral flexion
Lateral pelvic tilt (hip hitch)	Right hip abduction	Left lateral flexion
Forward rotation	Right hip MR	Rotation to the left
Backward rotation	Right hip LR	Rotation to the right

MR = medial rotation; LR = lateral rotation.

Reprinted, by permission, from C.C. Norkin and P.K. Levangie, 1992, *Joint structure and function: A comprehensive analysis*, 2d ed. (Philadelphia: Davis).

Controlling Spinal Range of Motion

If the trunk is moving slowly, a subject feels tissue tension at the end range and is able to stop a movement short of the full end range—thereby protecting the spinal tissues from overstretching. However, rapid trunk movements can build up sufficient momentum to push the spine to the full end range, thereby stressing the spinal tissues. Many amateur and even professional sports directors, teachers, and coaches have their charges engage in rapid and ballistic warm-up exercises, performed with high numbers of repetitions. These activities can lead to excessive flexibility and a reduction in passive stability of the spine.

THE MECHANICS OF LIFTING

Many individuals engage in some sort of lifting throughout the day. This section briefly describes the mechanical factors and the muscle work involved in lifting. See chapter 11 for proper lifting techniques.

Lifting As a Set of Torques

Lifting an object from the ground actually represents a rather complex mechanical problem. One must create a set of torques (technically, torque = force × distance to axis of rotation), involving both the body and the object to be lifted, that will produce the desired outcome (figure 2.15). The forces created during flexion by leverage, body weight, and muscle force—plus those created by the weight being lifted—must be overcome

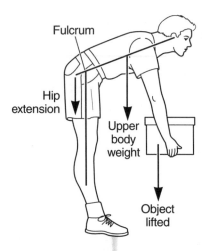

Fulcrum

Hip extension

Upper body weight

Object lifted

Figure 2.15 The mechanics of lifting.

by an opposing extension force created by the hip extensor muscles as they contract upon the spine.

• If the spine is not stable, posterior pelvic tilting brought about by the hip extensors (gluteus maximus and the hamstrings) merely increases the flexion of the spine.

• If the spine is stable, the power (created when the hip extensors posteriorly tilt the pelvis) is transmitted by the erector spinae along the length of the spine to the upper limb, which then delivers the force to the object being lifted.

The hip extensor muscles are better suited than the erector spinae to initiate a lift from a flexed position. A 150-pound athlete develops a torque of about 10,000 inch-pounds in lifting a 450-pound weight. Although the hip extensors can generate a torque of about 15,000 inch-pounds, the erector spinae can generate only 3,000, or 30% of that required to perform the lift (Farfan 1988). Note that the bulk of the muscles creating the force (gluteus maximus) are some distance from the limb controlling the movement (compare this arrangement with the fingers: the muscles that flex and extend the fingers are located not right above the fingers, where they would be in the way, but in the forearm). When prescribing exercises within the back stability program to help re-educate a person in correct lifting habits, emphasize use of the hip extensors (spinal extensors are far less important in this case), working *with a stable spine*. The hip hinge action, which emphasizes the gluteals, is a good exercise to use (see page 72).

Modeling the spine as a cantilever system according to standard mechanical principles, one can calculate the torques of various forces acting on the spine during lifting. Where the leverage is in equilibrium, the sum of the torques is zero, with flexion forces exactly balancing extension forces. It is possible to calculate both the force needed to lift an object and the resulting compression force on the lumbar spine (Sullivan 1997). In order to lift a weight, the muscles and connective tissues in the lumbar spine must counteract the flexion caused by the weight by providing an equal amount of extension (figure 2.15). However, since the weight is far from the fulcrum while the lower back muscles and tissues are very near to it, the muscles and tissues have much less leverage and must therefore exert much more force than just the weight of the object being lifted. Meanwhile, the vertebral joints experience a compression that is the sum of this force and the weight of the object. That sum is much greater than the weight alone and can be *very large indeed!* Yet, using postmortem measurements of actual vertebral strength, Perey (1957) estimated that lifting a weight heavier than 110 kg (242.5 lb.) would exceed the compressive strength of vertebrae. Such calculations clearly indicate that the *spinal column alone* cannot bear excessively large weights without undergoing severe damage. In order to reduce the compressive force acting on the spinal column when lifting large amounts of weight (as, for example, in Olympic weight lifting), an individual must substantially strengthen all the vertebral reinforcing mechanisms reviewed in chapter 3.

KEY POINT: The spinal column itself is not strong enough to bear the compression force from lifting heavy weights. The force created by the torque of lifting heavy weights can be many, many times the force of the weight itself—the muscles and connective tissues of the lumbar spine must bear the large majority of the forces involved. If these soft tissues are not sufficiently trained, severe injury can result.

The Flexion Relaxation Response in Lifting

When a subject flexes the spine during a lift, the erector spinae are electrically silent just short of full flexion (Kippers and Parker 1984). This phenomenon, called the *flexion relaxation response* or *critical point*, is the result of elastic recoil (rebound) of the posterior ligaments and musculature. This point does not occur in all individuals (see below) and occurs later in the range of motion when weights are carried (Bogduk and Twomey 1991). During the final stages of flexion and from 2-10° extension (Sullivan 1997), movement occurs by recoil of the stretched tissues rather than by active muscle work.

KEY POINT: During bending, the erector spinae are electrically silent just short of full flexion. This phenomenon is the "flexion relaxation response."

If the erector spinae are in spasm, chronic low back pain often obliterates the flexion relaxation response. Failure of the muscles to relax prevents adequate perfusion with fresh blood and can lead to local ischemic muscle pain. Interestingly, during a squat lift with the back perfectly straight, the latissimus dorsi contracts powerfully at the beginning of the lift—perhaps to initiate extension by pulling on the thoracolumbar fascia (McGill and Norman 1986; Sullivan 1997). With extremely heavy lifts of any type, as subjects flex forward to the point of electrical silence, the positions of the vertebrae suggest that they do not reach the point at which the ligaments would be loaded (i.e., stretched or tensioned greater than at rest) (Cholewicki and McGill 1992).

The electrical silence of the muscles and the anatomical alignment of the vertebral segments suggest that the final degrees of flexion as well as the first degrees of extension occur through elastic recoil of the spinal extensor muscles. The length/tension relationship in muscles (figure 2.16) shows that a muscle loses active tension as it is stretched—but even toward the end of the range of movement, there is little decrease in total tension since an increase in passive force (recoil, as happens with a stretched rubber band) largely makes up for the decrease in active contraction. As the spine returns from a fully flexed position, the ligaments may produce some 50 N · m of tension while the recoiling muscles produce 200 N · m. The combined extensor forces of the two passive systems represents the major component of the "posterior ligamentous system" supporting the spine (Bogduk and Twomey 1991).

Arch Model of the Spine

Instead of representing the spine as a cantilever system as just described, one can use the model of an arch (Aspden 1987, 1989). The ends (abutments) of the arch are provided caudally by the sacrum and cranially by a combination of bodyweight and muscular/ligamentous forces. The principle difference between a lever and an arch is that the lever is externally supported, whereas the arch is intrinsically stable. Any load positioned on the convex surface of the arch will create an internal thrust line that runs in a straight

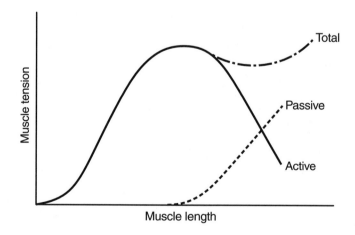

Figure 2.16 The length-tension relationship in muscles.
From Norris 1998.

line to the arch abutments (figure 2.17a). For the arch to remain stable, the thrust line must stay within the physical boundaries of the arch. The deeper within the arch the thrust line stays, the more stable the arch will be. In the case of the spine, the thrust line is positioned within the vertebral bodies.

Because a 100-kg weight lifted in a stooped position (lordosis lost) creates a thrust line outside the spine (figure 2.17b), the arch is unstable. By tensing the back extensor and abdominal muscles at the same time, however, one can create intra-abdominal pressure (IAP) that moves the thrust line back into the spine and increases spinal stability (figure 2.17c).

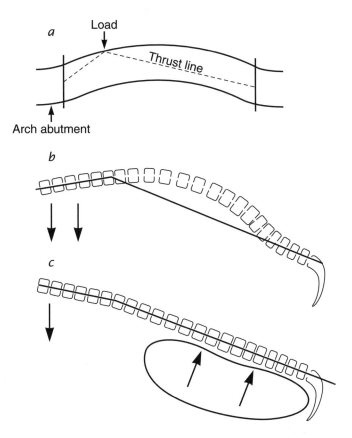

Figure 2.17 *(a)* General mechanics of an arch. A load on the convex surface of an arch creates an internal thrust line. For stability, the thrust line must stay within the depth of the arch ring. *(b)* Applying the arch model to the spine. Lifting a heavy weight in a stooped position creates a thrust line that moves outside the arch of the spine, making the spine unstable. *(c)* IAP acting on the anterior surface of the spine and adjustment of lordosis moves the thrust line back within the vertebral bodies.

Reprinted, by permission, from C. Norris, 1995, "Spinal stabilisation," *Physiotherapy Journal* 81(3): 4-12.

Moreover, an individual can use the spinal muscles (which are intrinsic to the arch) to adjust the lordosis, so that the thrust line continually remains within the arch of the spine. The stiffness of the spine (resistance to bending) also is increased through the thoracolumbar fascia (TLF) and hydraulic amplifier mechanisms.

Some writers believe the arch model of the spine seriously underestimates the compressive forces on the spine (Adams 1989). For further discussion of IAP and other stabilizing mechanisms, see chapter 3.

LIFTING METHODS

There are two basic ways to lift something: in the squat lift, a person bends the knees and back; in the stoop lift, the legs remain straight and the back alone bends. Because the legs are apart and bent with the squat lift, an individual can hold the object closer to the body's line of gravity—thereby reducing the length of the lever arm from the body's line of gravity to the center of gravity of the object. The disadvantage of the squat lift is that individuals are lifting more of their bodies (the legs and trunk as opposed to the trunk alone) and therefore must expend more energy than with a stoop lift. The erector spinae are more active in positions where the lordosis is maintained (Delitto et al. 1987)—after they have attained a fully erect position when lifting a heavy weight, people tend to lean back in order to balance the weight and to use their hip flexor muscles to resist further spinal extension and to stabilize their spines.

> **KEY POINT:** In a squat lift, a person can hold a weight closer to the body's center of gravity, thereby reducing the torque on the spine.

In addition to differentiating between the squat lift and stoop lift, we must also examine the difference between using a squat lift with the back lordotic (lumbar spine minimally extended) and with the back flat (lumbar spine minimally flexed). Lumbar curvature is calculated as the angle formed between the surface of the vertebral body of L1 and that of the sacrum (figure 2.18). The population mean value of this angle is 50°, although in children it is increased to 67° and in young males to as much as 74° (Bogduk and Twomey 1991) depending on posture type. The lordosis naturally results from the shapes of the vertebrae and disks of the lumbar spine. The L5-S1 vertebral disc is wedge shaped, its posterior height typically about 7 mm less than its anterior. The L5 vertebral body also is wedge shaped, its posterior height typically 3 mm less than its anterior. The remainder of the lordosis occurs because the discs themselves (not the vertebral bodies) are wedge shaped. The sacrum is angled at about 30° to the horizontal, and changes to this angle affect the sacroiliac joint.

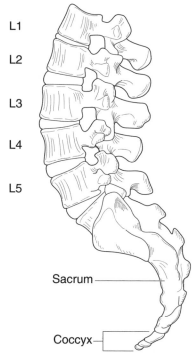

Figure 2.18 The curvature of the lumbar spine can be designated by the angle (Q) formed between lines through the surface of L1 and the sacrum.

Adapted, by permission, from J.K. Loudon, S.L. Bell, and J.M. Johnston, 1998, *The clinical orthopedic assessment guide* (Champaign, IL: Human Kinetics), 54.

Because the orientation of the vertebrae differ between the squat and stoop lifts, the load distribution is affected. The lengths of various trunk muscles also differ between the two lifts. Since the depth of the lumbar discs (6-12 mm) is considerably smaller than the vertical height of the lumbar vertebrae (30-45 mm), even minimal changes in vertebral angles can greatly deform the discs. A flexion angle of 10-12°, for example, stretches the posterior annulus by more than 50% (Adams and Dolan 1997). Repeated loading in a lordotic posture can cause compressive stress within the posterior annulus of a disc and load the adjacent facet joints. Maximal flexion (up to the elastic limit) can thin the posterior annulus and cause posterior prolapse. Minimal flexion (flatback), however, which brings the vertebral bodies into vertical alignment, equalizes compressive stress across the whole disc and unloads the facets (Adams et al. 1994). At 60-80% of maximum flexion, the posterior tissues exert a substantial extensor torque—yet there is only a small compression effect on the lumbar discs. Moreover, tension in the thoracolumbar fascia helps to stabilize the sacroiliac joint—and contraction of the gluteal muscles, the abdominals, and latissimus dorsi all increase the TLF tension in a flatback posture.

To lift a heavy object, one optimally should use a squat lift while maintaining the neutral position of the spine. The spine is likely to flatten as the weight is taken, and this technique should prevent hyperflexion as long as the object is pulled toward the pelvis.

KEY POINT: Have your client perform squat lifts when lifting an object, bringing the object in toward the pelvis. As your client begins to raise the weight, her lumbar spine flattens to minimally compress the lumbar discs and unload the facet joints. In this position, tissue recoil provides substantial extension power.

SUMMARY

- A spinal segment, comprising two adjacent vertebrae, is comparable to a simple leverage system, connected and held together by ligaments.

- Because spinal ligaments are interconnected with fasciae surrounding back muscles, which in turn eventually merge with ligaments and muscles as distant as the extremities of limbs, movements of most parts of the body can affect the stability of the spine.

- The deep abdominal muscles in particular are very important in keeping the spine stable (i.e., keeping vertebrae in line even during heavy lifting).

- Spinal discs, between each pair of vertebrae, absorb stress through stretching of the elastic fibers in the outer annulus and through cushioning by the highly plastic, hydrophilic nucleus pulposus. With age, the nucleus loses water content and the fibers lose elasticity.

- The facet joints are synovial joints between the inferior articular process of one vertebra and the superior articular process of its neighbor. Their articular cartilage can become brittle with age.

- Within the vertebra itself, compressive force is transmitted by both the cancellous (spongy) bone of the vertebral body and its cortical bone shell. Cancellous tissue declines with age. The vertebrae themselves, however, can bear only a small fraction of the load placed on the spine by heavy weights without experiencing serious injury.

- In order to successfully bear heavy weight, the spine must be stabilized by muscles and ligaments.

3

Stabilization Mechanisms in the Lumbar Spine

Devoid of its musculature, the human spine is inherently unstable. The spine of a fresh cadaver stripped of muscle can sustain a load of only 4-5 lb. before it buckles into flexion (Panjabi et al. 1989). Moreover, the center of gravity of the upper body (when standing upright) lies at sternal level (Norkin and Levangie 1992). This combination of flexibility and weight distribution is approximately comparable to balancing a 75-pound weight at the end of a 14-inch flexible rod (Farfan 1988).

From the strictly mechanical standpoint, discs don't contribute as much as one might think to the spine's strength: lifting heavy objects imposes on the lower lumbar spine a compressive force that greatly exceeds the failure load of the vertebral discs unless additional support is present (Bartelink 1957; Bradford and Spurling 1945; Morris et al. 1961).

By reducing the compression forces on lumbar discs, several mechanisms help stabilize the spine (Norris 1995a). These mechanisms, on which this chapter focuses, include the posterior ligamentous system, several processes involving the thoracolumbar fascia, actions of trunk muscles, and intra-abdominal pressure.

THE POSTERIOR LIGAMENTOUS SYSTEM

The interspinous and supraspinous ligaments, facet joint capsules, and thoracolumbar fascia (TLF) together provide passive support for the spine sufficient to balance between 24% and 55% of imposed flexion stress (Adams et al. 1980).

In the unstretched position, collagen fibers within the anterior and posterior longitudinal ligaments and the ligamentum flavum (see figure 2.3, page 16) are aligned haphazardly. When the ligaments are stretched as the spine flexes or extends, however, the collagen fibers become aligned and the ligament becomes stiffer (Hukins et al. 1990; Kirby et al. 1989). Prestressed by 10-13% at rest, the ligaments retract when cut (Hukins et al. 1990). The longitudinal ligaments therefore maintain a compressive force along the axis of the spine, causing it to act somewhat like a prestressed beam (Aspden 1992). The ligaments are viscoelastic (i.e., they stiffen when loaded rapidly). Rapid loading therefore increases the thrust within the spine and tends to approximate (bring closer together) the vertebrae, enhancing spinal stability.

Power created by the hip extensors posteriorly tilts the pelvis and is transmitted through the spine to the thorax and upper limbs via the ligamentous system. Some authors have maintained that for this passive mechanism to work, the spine must remain flexed. They argued that if the spine extends, tightness of the posterior ligaments will decrease and their ability to stabilize the spine will be lost (McGill and Norman 1986). More recently, however, it has been shown that the spine need not become kyphotic before it can create tension by stretching the tissues (Gracovetsky et al. 1990).

The posterior ligamentous system alone can sustain a maximum torque of only about 50 N · m (Bogduk and Twomey 1991), less than 25% of that of the contracting erector spinae. However, two passive systems are at work here (see page 38). In addition to the recoil from the posterior ligamentous sytem, the erector spinae are also recoiling. At the point of full flexion, these muscles no longer contract (they are electrically silent), but they do exert a force through recoil much like that of a giant elastic band. The force that the erector spinae create through recoil is about 200 N · m equal to their potential contractile force. The combined posterior musculoligamentous system therefore provides a substantial stabilizing mechanism in full flexion.

KEY POINT: The posterior ligaments of the spine can sustain 50 N · m of torque and resist over 50% of the flexion stress imposed on the spine. The passive tension (elastic recoil) in the stretched erector spinae can create 200 N · m of torque, equal to their maximum contraction.

THE THORACOLUMBAR FASCIA

The thoracolumbar fascia performs a number of important functions during back stability, which I briefly review here. Note that the fascia also acts to stabilize the sacroiliac joints.

Structure of the Thoracolumbar Fascia

The thoracolumbar (lumbardorsal) fascia (TLF) has three layers that cover the muscles of the back (figure 3.1). The anterior layer derives from fascia covering the quadratus lumborum and attaches to the transverse processes

> ## Terms You Should Know
>
> **aponeurosis** connective tissue that attaches muscle to bone
>
> **approximate (verb)** to move or bring objects closer together
>
> **contralateral** originating in or affecting the opposite side of the body
>
> **fascicle** a small bundle of nerve or muscle fibers
>
> **hoop pressure** the inward pressure exerted by the muscles surrounding the trunk
>
> **ipsilateral** on the same side (of the body)
>
> **kyphotic** convex curvature of the thoracic spine creating a hunchback
>
> **lamina** a thin flat layer or membrane
>
> **raphe, lateral** a ridge along the side of the erector spinae muscles formed by the connective tissue of the latissimus dorsi, internal obliques, and transversus abdominus

(Bogduk and Twomey 1991). The middle layer, behind the quadratus lumborum, attaches both to the transverse processes and to the intertransverse ligaments. Laterally, it extends to cover transversus abdominis. The posterior layer, which envelops the erector spinae, attaches from the spinous processes and wraps around the back muscles to blend with the rest of the TLF laterally to the iliocostalis. The point at which the layers blend is the lateral raphe.

The superficial layer of the TLF is continuous with the latissimus dorsi and gluteus maximus. Sometimes a few fibers attach to parts of the external oblique and trapezius, and some cross the body midline (Vleeming et al. 1995). At L4-L5 level, fibers from latissimus dorsi and gluteus maximus differ in orientation, giving the superficial layer of the TLF a crosshatched appearance. This appearance may even extend down to the L5-S2 level (Vleeming et al. 1997). The fibers of the deep layer are continuous with the sacrotuberous ligament (and through it to the biceps femoris muscle of the upper leg); and they attach to the posterior superior iliac spines, the iliac crests, and the sacroiliac ligaments (see figure 2.8, page 23). In the thoracic region, fibers of the serratus posterior inferior are continuous with the TLF (figure 3.2).

Thoracolumbar Fascia Mechanism

In addition to its passive role, the TLF has two further capacities that involve muscle contraction. The transversus abdominis, through its attachment to the lateral raphe, pulls on the TLF. Although both attach to the lateral raphe (figure 3.3), the deep laminae of the TLF angle upward, while

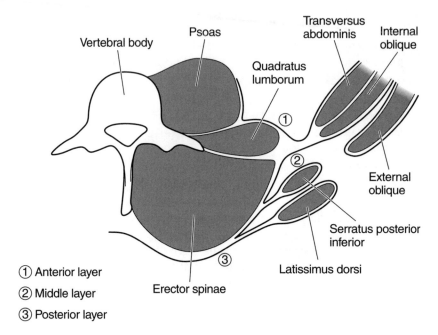

Figure 3.1 Cross section of trunk showing thoracolumbar fascia (TLF).

① Anterior layer
② Middle layer
③ Posterior layer

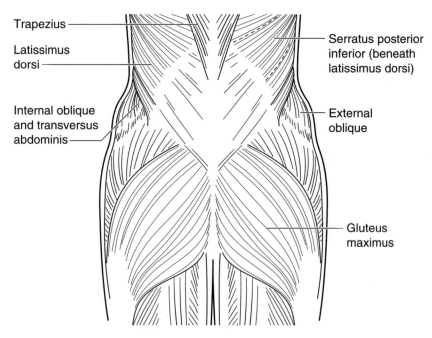

Figure 3.2 Muscle attachments into the thoracolumbar fascia (TLF).

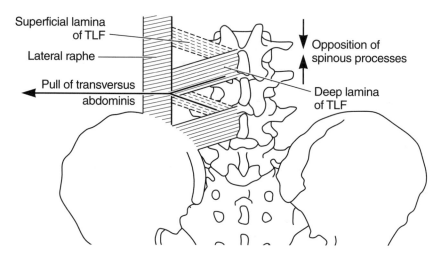

Figure 3.3 The thoracolumbar fascia mechanism. Through its attachment to the lateral raphe, the transversus abdominis pulls on the TLF. The angulation of both the deep and superficial layers of the TLF creates a net force that tends to approximate the vertebrae.

the superficial laminae angle downward. As the transversus abdominis contracts and pulls on the lateral raphe, the deep and superficial fibers of the TLF pull laterally for the most part, although some force is transmitted along the length of the TLF.

Originally, this approximating force was calculated as 57% of the force applied to the lateral raphe (Macintosh and Bogduk 1987), an increase in force termed the "gain" of the TLF (Gracovetsky et al. 1985). However, more detailed anatomical investigation has revealed that the torque created by contraction of transversus abdominis onto the TLF is between 3.9 and 5.9 N · m—compared to that from the back extensors of 250-280 N · m (Macintosh et al. 1987). Rather than actively extending the spine through the approximating force represented by "gain," then, the primary importance of the TLF seems to be providing passive resistance to flexion.

Thoracolumbar Fascia as Hydraulic Amplifier

The TLF exerts an even greater stabilizing effect through its role in the so-called hydraulic amplifier effect (Gracovetsky et al. 1977). The posterior layer of the TLF is retinacular tissue (i.e., very strong reinforcing connective tissue) that envelops the erector spinae. As the erector spinae contract, the TLF resists the expansion of the bellies of the shortening muscles by increasing tension in the fascia. Some believe that the predominant antiflexion effect of the TLF occurs via this hydraulic amplifier effect rather than by its pull on the transversus abdominis (Macintosh et al. 1987). Restriction of the radial expansion of the erector spinae by the TLF has been shown to increase the stress generated by these muscles by as much as 30% (Hukins et al. 1990).

Thoracolumbar Fascia Coupling and the Sacroiliac Joint

A combination of form closure and force closure stabilizes the sacroiliac joint (SIJ) (Vleeming et al. 1990). **Form closure** arises from the anatomical alignment of the bones of the ilium and sacrum, where the sacrum forms a kind of keystone between the wings of the pelvis (Norris 1998). **Force closure** results from muscles pulling laterally onto fascia and ligaments that pass over the joint. The combination of form and force closure creates a very useful self-locking mechanism within the SIJ. Any activity that weakens these forms of closure can create pathological symptoms in the SIJ.

Nutation (see table 2.2 on page 24) tensions the SIJ ligaments, pulling the posterior parts of the iliac bones together and increasing SIJ compression. Two ligaments are of special importance to self locking—the *sacrotuberous ligament* connecting the sacrum to the ischial tuberosity, and the *long dorsal sacroiliac ligament* from the third and fourth sacral segments to the posterior superior iliac spines (PSIS). Both ligaments blend over the posterolateral aspect of the sacrum to form an expansion approximately 20 mm wide and 60 mm long. The ligaments attach to the posterior layer of the TLF and to the aponeurosis of the erector spinae. Nutation tensions the sacrotuberous ligament, while counternutation tensions the long dorsal sacroiliac (SI) ligament. The SI ligament is tensioned by contraction of the biceps femoris and of the gluteus maximus.

Force closure of the SIJ opens the possibility of treating SIJ lesions with exercise therapy either passively (automobilization) or actively through contraction of the biceps femoris, gluteus maximus, latissimus dorsi, or erector spine. Clearly, if muscle affects the SIJ, as has been shown by Vleeming's work (Vleeming et al. 1995a), training these muscles could improve SIJ functions. Moreover, any muscle that tensions the TLF should also affect force closure of the SIJ.

When the erector spinae contract, they pull the sacrum forward—inducing nutation of the SIJ and tensing the interosseous and sacrotuberous ligaments. The iliac portion of the muscle tends to pull the cranial aspect of the SIJ together, whereas the action of nutation pulls the caudal aspect apart. The gluteus maximus can compress the SIJ directly and indirectly through its attachment to the sacrotuberous ligament. This occurs particularly when the gluteus maximus contracts with the contralateral latissimus dorsi and both muscles tension the TLF, whose fibers join the two muscles. Tension in the sacrotuberous ligament is increased by tensioning the long head of biceps femoris. This occurs most noticeably in a flexed trunk or stooped position, in which the sacrotuberous ligament is also tensioned by the sacral portion of the erector spinae and the gluteus maximus.

SIJ pain frequently occurs during and after pregnancy, when laxness of the SIJ ligaments reduces form closure of the joints. Female gymnasts experience similar problems: the inherent hyperflexibility of gymnastics generally increases the laxity of the pelvic ligaments, reducing the form closure that they produce. The increased muscular stability resulting from the muscular demands of the sport is compensated for by the laxness, as long as the women continue their activity. When their muscle strength declines after they stop practicing the sport, the SIJ is left unstable and open to pathology. SIJ pain of this type is often helped by using a pelvic belt; it may also be helped by improving force closure of the SIJ by using stabilization techniques for the lumbar spine and enhancing gluteal muscle strength using the hip hinge action (see page 77).

> **KEY POINT:** ▸ Specific exercise can improve stability of the sacroiliac joint by restoring the natural mechanisms of form closure and force closure.

TRUNK MUSCLE ACTION

Facilitating co-contraction of the muscles surrounding the lumbar spine—including the erector spinae, transversus abdominis, multifidus, and the oblique abdominals—may enhance spinal stability (Richardson et al. 1990).

Spinal Extensor Muscles

The spinal extensors may be broadly categorized into *superficial* muscles (the erector spinae) that travel the length of the lumbar spine and attach to the sacrum and pelvis, and *deep*, or intersegmental (unisegmental) muscles (multifidi, interspinales, and intertransversarii) that span the spaces between the individual lumbar segments.

The intersegmental muscles, being more deeply placed, are closer to the center of rotation of the spine and have a shorter lever arm than the superficial muscles. However, their closeness to the center of rotation means that the change in length of intersegmental muscles is less for any given change in the spine's angular position; and the muscles' shorter length gives them a faster reaction time, creating a smoother and more efficient stabilizing control system (Panjabi et al. 1989). The intersegmental nature of these muscles also means that they are able to "fine tune" the spinal movements by acting on individual lumbar segments rather than the whole spine (Aspden 1992).

Being larger in size and further from the center of rotation, the superficial muscles are better placed to create gross sagittal rotation movements, while the intersegmental muscles are of greater importance to spinal stability (Panjabi et al. 1989). Furthermore, because the smaller intersegmental muscles have about seven times the number of muscle spindles (Bastide et al. 1989) than the larger muscles have, they have a greater proprioceptive role (see following discussion).

Deep (Intersegmental) Muscles

Of the deeply placed intersegmental muscles, the multifidus is most important for lumbar stability. The fibers of multifidus are arranged segmentally, and each fascicle of a given vertebra has a separate innervation by the medial branch of the dorsal ramus of the vertebra below (Macintosh and Bogduk 1986). The primary function of each multifidus fascicle may be to control lordosis at its particular vertebral level and to independently counteract any imposed loading (Aspden 1992). The action of the multifidus can be resolved into a small horizontal and very much larger vertical component (figure 3.4), which (as is clear when viewed from the side) acts at 90° to the spinous processes. This configuration enables multifidus to produce posterior sagittal rotation (rocking) of the lumbar vertebrae (Macintosh and Bogduk 1986). This action neutralizes spinal flexion caused as a secondary action when the oblique abdominals produce spinal rotation. Because the line of action of the long fascicles of multifidus lies behind the lumbar spine, the muscle also increases lumbar lordosis. Multifidus is active through the whole range of flexion, during rotation in either direction, and during extension movements of the hip (Valencia and Munro 1985). Posterior sagittal rotation occurs during all flexion movements, in order to resist the anterior sagittal rotation

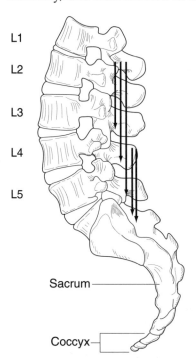

Figure 3.4 Lateral view showing the line of action of multifidus, with its vertical alignment.

Adapted, by permission, from J.K. Loudon, S.L. Bell, and J.M. Johnston, 1998, *The clinical orthopedic assessment guide* (Champaign, IL: Human Kinetics), 54.

that naturally accompanies flexion. The importance of multifidus in producing this action is therefore essential to stability of the lumbar spine in normal movements.

Panjabi's (1992) description of instability (as a reduction in stiffness within the neutral zone of the lumbar spine) is particularly relevant to multifidus function. Multifidus is a muscle well positioned to enhance segmental stiffness in the neutral zone and contributes nearly 70% of the stiffness resulting from muscle contraction (Wilke et al. 1995).

Real-time ultrasound imaging has revealed marked asymmetry of the multifidus in patients with low back pain (Hides et al. 1994). Cross-sectional area (CSA) of the multifidus was markedly reduced on the ipsilateral side to symptoms, the site of reduction corresponding to the level of lumbar lesion as assessed by manual therapy palpation. The muscle also showed a rounder shape, suggesting muscle spasm. The suggested mechanism for the CSA reduction was by inhibition through perceived pain via a long loop reflex. The level of vertebral pathology may have been targeted to protect the damaged tissues from movement. The authors suggested that the rapid muscle wasting (less than 14 days in 20 of the 26 patients studied) may have resulted from spasm-induced reduction in circulation to the muscle.

In addition to changes in muscle bulk, Biedermann et al. (1991) observed altered fiber types in the multifidus of low back pain (LBP) patients; patients who tended to decrease their physical and social activities as a result of LBP showed a reduced ratio of slow twitch to fast twitch muscle fibers. This could be the muscle's adaptive response to changes in functional demand placed on it, and/or the injury may have caused a shift in recruitment patterns of motor units of the paraspinal muscles, with the fast twitch motor units being recruited before the slow twitch units. Pathologic changes in the multifidus following low back pain include a moth-eaten appearance of type I fibers (Hides et al. 1996) and an increase in fatty deposits (Parkkola et al. 1993).

Recovery of multifidus function following low back pain does not occur automatically following the resolution of pain and resumption of normal daily activity. In a study comparing medical treatment alone (1-3 days' bed rest, analgesics, and anti-inflammatory medication) with medical treatment plus specific exercise therapy to the multifidus, Hides et al. (1996) showed that multifidus activity could be retrained. Subjects who had experienced first-episode acute low back pain showed an average of 24% reduction in CSA to the multifidus on the painful side. The difference between painful and painless sides changed from nearly 17% after 4 weeks to 14% after 10 weeks in those subjects receiving medical treatment alone. For those who received additional exercise therapy, however, the mean values were 0.7% at 4 weeks dropping to 0.24% after 10 weeks (figure 3.5).

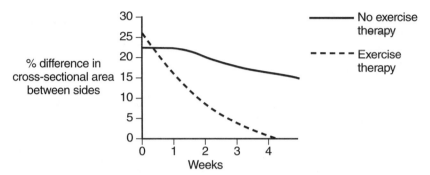

Figure 3.5 Ultrasound imaging results of multifidus muscle recovery.
Reprinted from Hides et al. 1996.

KEY POINT: Low back pain leads to reduced cross-sectional area in the multifidus muscle. As the pain reduces, recovery is not automatic—rehabilitation is required.

Superficial Muscles

The **lumbar erector spinae** consists of two muscles: the iliocostalis and the longissimus (figure 3.6). Each of these muscles has two components arising from both the thoracic and lumbar spine. Functionally, therefore, the erector spinae can be considered in four distinct groups: lumbar longissimus, lumbar iliocostalis, thoracic longissimus, and thoracic iliocostalis (Macintosh and Bogduk 1987).

The force produced by the **lumbar longissimus** can be resolved into a large vertical vector and a smaller horizontal vector (figure 3.7). However, the fascicle attachments are closer to the axis of sagittal rotation than those of multifidus, so their effect on posterior sagittal rotation is less. Because the horizontal vectors of lumbar longissimus are directed backward, the muscle is able to draw the vertebrae backward into posterior translation and restore the anterior

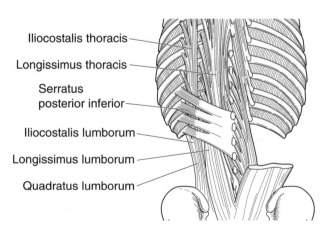

Iliocostalis thoracis

Longissimus thoracis

Serratus posterior inferior

Iliocostalis lumborum

Longissimus lumborum

Quadratus lumborum

Figure 3.6 Muscles of the back.

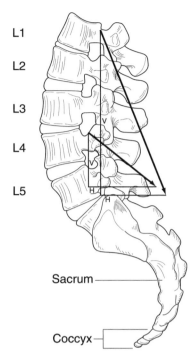

L1
L2
L3
L4
L5
Sacrum
Coccyx

Figure 3.7 Lateral view of the lumbar spine, showing the line of the lumbar iliocostalis and lumbar longissimus, and their more oblique orientation. Note the greater horizontal force vector (H) and smaller verical force vector (V) of the lower fibers of these muscles.

Adapted, by permission, from J.K. Loudon, S.L. Bell, and J.M. Johnston, 1998, *The clinical orthopedic assessment guide* (Champaign, IL: Human Kinetics), 54.

translation that occurs with lumbar flexion. The upper lumbar fascicles are better equipped to facilitate posterior sagittal rotation, whereas the lower levels are better suited to resist anterior translation.

The **lumbar iliocostalis** has a similar action to that of the lumbar longissimus. In addition, the muscle cooperates with multifidus to neutralize flexion caused when the abdominals rotate the trunk.

The **thoracic longissimus** can indirectly increase lumbar lordosis via its effect on the aponeurosis of the erector spinae. It also indirectly laterally flexes the lumbar spine through its lateral flexion of the thoracic spine.

The **thoracic iliocostalis** attaches not to the lumbar vertebrae but to the iliac crest. On contraction, these fascicles increase lordosis; through their additional leverage from the ribs, they indirectly laterally flex the lumbar spine. During contralateral rotation, the ribs separate, stretching the thoracic iliocostalis which can therefore act as a limiting factor to this movement. On contraction, the thoracic iliocostalis will de-rotate the rib cage and lumbar spine from a position of contralateral rotation.

It is probably the endurance rather than the strength of the erector spinae that is important to LBP rehabilitation. Endurance has been used as a predictor for susceptibility to LBP (Beiring-Sorensen 1984). Moreover, subjects with a history of LBP may have reduced endurance of the back extensors compared to normal subjects, but similar strength (Jorgensen and Nicolaisen 1987). As fatigue increases, subjects with LBP show reduced precision and control of trunk movements. Loss of torque from the trunk muscles in these subjects is relatively less than the loss of control and precision (Parnianpour et al. 1988), indicating that a rehabilitation program should include restoration of endurance for the spinal extensors. Selective recruitment of the torque-producing superficial muscles from the stabilizing deep muscles is also important for rehabilitation of active lumbar stabilization (Ng and Richardson 1994).

The **quadratus lumborum** (figure 3.6) can be an important back stabilizer in certain circumstances (McGill et al. 1996). The muscle lies deeper than the erector spinae and has medial and lateral fibers. The medial fibers connect the lumbar transverse processes to the ilium and iliolumbar ligament or the 12th rib, while the lateral fibers directly connect the ilium and iliolumbar ligament and 12th rib (Bogduk and Twomey 1991). The quadratus lumborum has a small extensor torque and a larger lateral flexion torque and is able to stabilize the lumbar spine via its segmental attachments (McGill et al. 1996). EMG with fine wire electrodes has shown the muscle to be more active during lateral bending than during extension and especially active in upright standing and unilateral carrying (McGill et al. 1996). Side-support actions shift some of the loading of the muscles from the discs and facet joints of the lumbar spine to the side (McGill 1998). This role of the quadratus lumborum as a potential stabilizer of the lumbar spine expands the traditionally recognized role of the muscle as a prime mover of side flexion and as an auxiliary muscle of respiration.

The Iliopsoas

The **iliopsoas** (figure 3.8) consists of the separate psoas and iliacus muscles. The psoas major arises from the vertebral bodies and discs of the lumbar and 12th thoracic vertebrae and from their transverse processes. The muscle passes downward and laterally, beneath the inguinal ligament, to blend with the fibers of iliacus and then to attach onto the posterior aspect of the lesser trochanter of the femur. The iliacus is a large triangular muscle on the anterior aspect of the pelvis. It arises primarily from the upper and posterior portions of the iliac fossa, but some fibers have been found on the sacrum and anterior sacroiliac ligament (Palastanga et al. 1994). The fibers from iliacus pass downward and medially to blend with those of psoas major and attach into the lesser trochanter, a few fibers merging with the joint capsule.

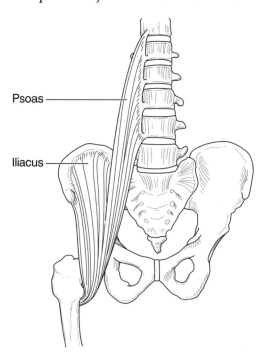

Psoas

Iliacus

Figure 3.8 The iliopsoas muscle, comprising the psoas and the iliacus, anterior view.

The iliopsoas flexes the hip; with the hip fixed, it anteriorly tilts the pelvis and flexes the lumbar spine. Although these actions are minimal, the psoas major extends the upper lumbar spine and flexes the lower lumbar spine (Bogduk et al. 1992); far more important is its production of compression and shear forces over the lumbar spine. The individual fascicles of psoas spiral anteromedially and are all of similar lengths. The lines of action of these fascicles run very close to the axis of rotation of the lumbar spine, giving the muscle fascicles very small torque arms and reducing the muscle's ability to flex the trunk on the stationary hip. However, the compression and shear forces created by the psoas on the lumbar spine are considerable and may even equal full trunk weight. The shearing force exerted on L5-S1 by maximum contraction of a single psoas muscle is nearly twice that exerted on this joint by trunk weight in normal upright standing (Bogduk et al. 1992). Because the two components of iliopsoas have a separate innervation (psoas from the anterior rami and L1-3, and iliacus from the femoral nerve), they can be activated separately. In a study using fine wire electrodes guided by high-resolution ultrasound, Andersson et al. (1995) showed selective recruitment of iliacus during contralateral leg extension from single-leg standing. No postural activity was seen in either muscle during relaxed standing or with the whole trunk flexed to 30°. When the contralateral hand was loaded (34-kg weight), psoas was active but iliacus was electrically silent. During sitting with a straight back, psoas was active but iliacus relatively silent; while in relaxed sitting, both muscles were inactive. Both muscles showed moderate activity when subjects sat with an anteriorly tilted pelvis and an increased lordosis. During abdominal exercise, both muscles were active during straight-leg sit-ups—with even higher activity during sit-ups with the knees and hips flexed to 90° (crunch position). However, little activity was seen when subjects performed trunk curls from the crunch position. During straight-leg raising, both muscles were active when the ipsilateral leg was lifted; both were inactive when the contralateral leg lifted (table 3.1).

Abdominal Muscles

The abdominal muscle group consists of four muscles, divided into two groups. The *deep* (anterolateral) abdominals are transversus abdominis and internal oblique; the *superficial* (front) abdominals are the rectus abdominis and external oblique.

Anatomy of the Superficial Abdominals

The **rectus abdominis** (figure 3.9) is positioned vertically at the front of the abdomen. It attaches from the symphasis pubis and pubic crest and runs to the xiphoid process and 5/6/7th ribs, being broader superiorly. The lateral border (semilunaris) can be seen in lean subjects, as can the central separation between the two muscles, the linea alba. Of the three

Table 3.1 Psoas and Iliacus Activity Measured on EMG As a Percentage of Maximum

Starting position	Psoas %	Iliacus %
Single-leg standing	0	0
Same-leg flexion (90°)	99	99
Opposite-leg extension (30°)	0	26
Same-leg abduction	36	56
Standing	0	0
Standing with trunk flexed to 30°	0	0
Standing opposite hand loaded	11	0
Sitting with straight back	9	4
Relaxed sitting	0	0
Sitting, hyperlordosis and pelvic tilt	17	22
Sit-up, straight legs	52	42
Sit-up, legs 45° to floor	88	60
Trunk curl, legs straight	0	0
Trunk curl, legs 90° (end range)	4	0
Straight-leg, raising (bilateral)	59	58

Data from Andersson et al. 1995.

noticeable tendinous intersections of this muscle, one is level with the umbilicus, one is level with the xiphoid, and one is midway between the two. Each rectus muscle is enclosed within a fibrous sheath (the rectus sheath) formed from the aponeuroses of the internal and external oblique muscles and of the transversus abdominis. These aponeuroses join centrally to form the linea alba. The rectus sheath changes at a level midway between the pubic symphasis and the umbilicus. In the upper area of the muscle, above this point, the aponeurosis of internal oblique splits into two, one part passing behind the rectus and the other in front. The aponeurosis of transversus abdominis fuses with the posterior portion of the sheath, while the aponeurosis of external oblique fuses with the anterior sheath. In the lower portion of the muscle (below the midpoint between the pubis and umbilicus), the oblique abdominal and transversus abdominis aponeuroses pass in front of the rectus, and as a result the rectus is less visible in this region (Palastanga et al. 1994).

The **external oblique** (figure 3.9) is positioned on the anterolateral aspect of the abdomen, with its fibers running downward and medially. It attaches from the outer borders of the lower eight ribs (and their costal cartilages) and then passes toward the midline. The muscle interdigitates

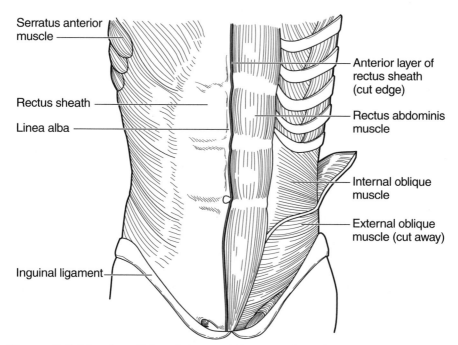

Serratus anterior muscle

Rectus sheath

Linea alba

Inguinal ligament

Anterior layer of rectus sheath (cut edge)

Rectus abdominis muscle

Internal oblique muscle

External oblique muscle (cut away)

Figure 3.9 Muscles of the abdomen I (intermediate dissection).

with the serratus anterior (above) and latissimus dorsi (below). The lateral fibers are almost vertical and attach to the iliac crest, while the medial fibers attach into the rectus sheath. The lower border of the muscle aponeurosis passes between the pubic tubercle and the anterior superior iliac spine to form the inguinal ligament.

Anatomy of the Deep Abdominals

The **internal oblique** (figure 3.9) is deep to the external oblique and attaches from the lateral two-thirds of the inguinal ligament and the anterior two-thirds of the iliac crest. It also takes attachment from the thoracolumbar fascia. The fibers fan outward and upward (the posterior fibers being almost vertical) to attach to the inferior borders of the lower four ribs. The anterior fibers pass medially to help form the rectus sheath (figure 3.10). The portion of the muscle that attaches to the inguinal ligament joins its neighboring fibers from transversus abdominis to form the conjoint tendon.

The **transversus abdominis** (figure 3.10) is the deepest of the sheet-like abdominal muscles and attaches from the lateral third of the inguinal ligament and the anterior two-thirds of the inner lip of the iliac crest (Palastanga et al. 1994). In addition, it has an attachment from the thoracolumbar fascia (where it merges with internal oblique to form the lateral raphe) and

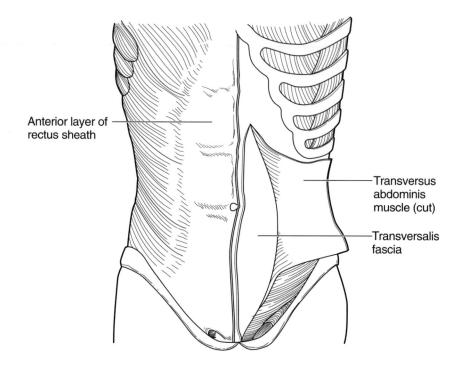

Figure 3.10 Muscles of the abdomen II (deep dissection).

from the lower six ribs, where it interdigitates with the diaphragm. Its fibers pass horizontally to merge into the rectus sheath (figure 3.11), with the lower fibers attaching to the inguinal ligament and merging with the fibers of the internal oblique to form the conjoint tendon. The lower part of the transversus abdominis forms into the transversalis fascia in which lies the deep inguinal ring.

Functions of the Abdominals

The rectus abdominis and lateral fibers of external oblique are the prime movers of trunk flexion; the internal oblique and transversus abdominis are the major stabilizers (Miller and Medeiros 1987). The rectus and external oblique are superficial muscles that often dominate trunk actions. The transversus and internal oblique are more deeply placed, and patients often are unable to contract them voluntarily.

The rectus abdominis flexes the trunk by approximating the pelvis and rib cage. EMG investigation has shown that trunk flexion emphasizes the supraumbilical portion, whereas posterior pelvic tilt shows greater activity in the infraumbilical portion (Guimaraes et al.

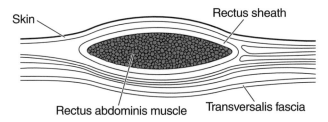

Figure 3.11 Cross section of the rectus sheath.

1991; Lipetz and Gutin 1970). Abdominal hollowing activates the internal oblique and transversus muscles (Richardson et al. 1992), and the transversus acts at the initiation of movement to stabilize the trunk in overhead and lower-limb actions (Hodges and Richardson 1996).

In resisted actions such as sport or lifting, the abdominal muscles essentially function to stabilize the trunk and provide a firm base of support for the arms and legs to work against. If stability is poor (in relation to total power of the subject), some of the energy of the limb actions can displace the pelvis and trunk instead of providing the desired limb movement. Compare what would happen if a baseball batter wearing sneakers were standing on ice when he connected with the ball, rather than having his feet dug into firm ground—much of the energy of the swing would be lost, and his body would twist awkwardly. In the same way, if trunk stability is poor, limb power suffers and additional stress is placed on the spinal tissues if they move to full end range.

Consider an overhead lifting action performed with an unstable spine (figure 3.12, a and b): if the pelvis tilts forward, lumbar lordosis increases and the abdominal muscles overstretch as the lumbar spine moves into full extension (see page 34). In this case, what trunk stability is present comes from facet joint approximation and elastic recoil of noncontractile tissues (passive stability) rather than from muscle action (active stability) (see

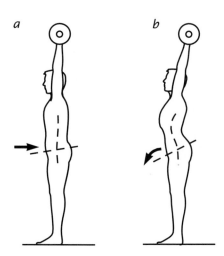

Figure 3.12 Trunk stability in overhead lifting: *(a)* active stability of the trunk through tight abdominals and level pelvis, resulting in reduced stress on lumbar tissues; *(b)* passive stability of the trunk through lax abdominals and tilted pelvis, resulting in increased stress on lumbar tissues.

From C. Norris, 1998, *Diagnosis and management*, 2d ed. (Oxford: Butterworth Heinemann), 175. Reprinted by permission of Butterworth Heinemann Publishers, a division of Reed Educational & Professional Publishing Ltd.

page 30). The fundamental key to safe and effective abdominal training in sport is to train for trunk stability before training for trunk muscle performance. In this way, the exercises are performed on a spine made stable by muscle rather than placing excessive stress on spinal joints before muscle stability has had time to build up.

> **KEY POINT:** ▶ Stability forms the foundation of all trunk exercise. Individuals should train for trunk stability *before* training for muscle performance.

Patterns of Coordination Among the Abdominals During Spinal Movement

In terms of spinal stabilization, the contraction speed of the abdominals is more critical than their strength when they react to a force tending to displace the lumbar spine (Saal and Saal 1989). Moreover, the ability of a patient to dissociate deep abdominal function from that of the superficial abdominals is important, and the key to lumbar stabilization appears to be the *ratio* rather than the *intensity* of muscle activity. Abdominal hollowing (rather than a sit-up movement) works the transversus abdominis and internal oblique (not the rectus abdominis and the external oblique) (Richardson et al. 1992). Patients with chronic low back pain (CLBP) are poorer at using the internal oblique than the rectus abdominis and external oblique, reflecting a shift in the pattern of motor activity (O'Sullivan et al. 1997). As CLBP patients attempt an abdominal hollowing action, they tend to substitute the superficial muscles that override the deep abdominals. When expressed as a ratio of internal oblique over rectus abdominis (IO/RA), the value from the control group (non-LBP) was 8.74 while the CLBP group had a ratio of only 2.41—indicating a much larger proportional contribution to hollowing by the internal oblique in the control group (figure 3.13). Pain inhibition in

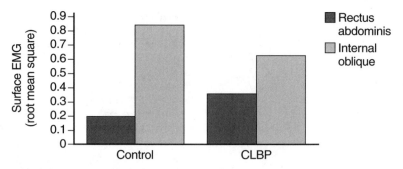

Figure 3.13 Abdominal muscle activation in chronic low back pain (CLBP). Data from O'Sullivan et al. 1997.

the subjects with CLBP may have led to altered muscle recruitment and compensatory strategies (O'Sullivan et al. 1997).

EMG measurements of trunk muscles have shown that the muscles do not simply work as prime movers of the spine but show antagonistic activity during various movements. The oblique abdominals are more active than predicted, to help stabilize the trunk. In a study by Zetterberg et al. (1987), subjects' abdominal muscle activities during maximum trunk extension ranged from 32% to 68% of their longissimus activities. As would be expected, the ipsilateral muscles showed maximum activity in resisted lateral flexion—but the contralateral muscles were also active at about 10-20% of the maximum values.

The coordinated patterns among the abdominal muscles are task-specific. But the *only* muscle that is active in all patterns is the transversus abdominis. During maximum voluntary isometric trunk extension, transversus abdominis is the only one of the abdominal muscles to show marked activity. It is also the muscle most consistently related to changes in intra-abdominal pressure (IAP) (Cresswell et al. 1992). The transversus abdominis not only contracts whenever the trunk moves in any direction—its activity always *precedes* the contraction of the other trunk muscles *in the normal (non-LBP) subject* (Cresswell et al. 1994).

> **KEY POINT:**▶ Transversus abdominis is the only abdominal muscle to be active in trunk movements in all directions. Its activity always precedes that of the other abdominal muscles in normal subjects.

When people engage in repeated movements, their bodies *anticipate* the predictable load and the muscles brace themselves accordingly. Using fine wire electrodes, Hodges and Richardson (1996) assessed abdominal muscle action during 10 repetitions of shoulder flexion, extension, and abduction. They found that transversus abdominis contracted before the shoulder muscles by as much as 38.9 milliseconds. The reaction time for the deltoid was on average 188 msec, with the abdominal muscles (except transversus) following the deltoid contraction by 9.84 msec. With subjects who had a history of low back pain, however, the contraction of the transversus failed to precede that of the deltoid, indicating that the subjects had *lost the anticipatory nature of stability* (figure 3.14). These highly significant data reveal a uniform dysfunction in the motor control of transversus abdominis in people with low back pain—the problem is not simply one of muscle strength. It appears that the anticipatory nature of transversus may be lost in those with low back pain, leaving open the possibility that this mechanism may be redeveloped therapeutically.

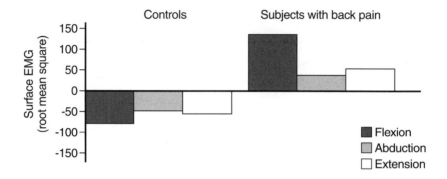

Figure 3.14 Activity of transversus abdominis muscle during shoulder movements. Note that subjects with back pain had a longer transversus reaction time. Point 0 represents the onset of shoulder movement.

KEY POINT: Patients with chronic low back pain exhibit a motor control deficit (alteration in muscle reaction timing and anticipatory bracing) in the transversus abdominis.

A number of authors have highlighted contraction of the abdominal muscles before the initiation of limb movement as an example of a feed-forward postural reaction (Friedli et al. 1984; Aruin and Latach 1995). In these cases, as would be expected, the erector spinae and the external oblique contract before arm flexion, while the rectus abdominis contracts before arm extension. In each case, the trunk muscles act to limit the reactive body movement toward the moving limb. Contraction of the transversus before the other abdominal muscle has been described by Cresswell et al. (1994) in response to trunk movements, but anticipatory contraction during limb movements is a newer finding. The transversus abdominis seems to be contracting during posture not simply to bring the body back closer to the posture line but to increase the stiffness of the lumbar region and enhance stability (Hodges et al. 1996).

INTRA-ABDOMINAL PRESSURE MECHANISM

Intra-abdominal pressure (IAP) is sometimes described as *intratruncal pressure* (Watkins 1999), although the latter term includes both intra-abdominal and intrathoracic pressure. Intrathoracic pressure is created during inspiration by expanding the lungs within the ribcage to coincide with a lift or other effort. Although intrathoracic pressure can be useful in competitive sport, I do not emphasize it within this text because the rather complex coordination between it and abdominal hollowing (described later) makes it unsuitable for most rehabilitation programs. Timing inspiration with effort, moreover, can lead to use of the Valsalva maneuver where the breath is held to maintain increased intrathoracic pressure. If done during exercise, the Valsalva can raise blood pressure to dangerous levels (Linsenbardt et al. 1992), an inappropriate situation given the poor health status of many individuals with back pain.

IAP involves synchronous contraction of the abdominal muscles, the diaphragm, and the muscles of the pelvic floor. The deep abdominals (transversus abdominis and internal oblique) are the more important of the abdominal muscle groups in this respect since they are visceral compressors rather than flexors. Although they have no name for it, most people experience IAP in everyday life—as, for example, when the muscles contract reflexively to defend the abdomen from a direct blow. The theoretical basis for the IAP mechanism is that pressure within the abdomen, acting against the pelvis and diaphragm, provides additional extensor torque to the spine (figure 3.15)—moreover, the "inflated balloon" acts on a torque arm that is as much as three times greater than that of the erector spinae.

KEY POINT: Intra-abdominal pressure is created by synchronous contraction of the abdominal muscles, the diaphragm, and the muscles of the pelvic floor.

Contraction of the transversus abdominis and the internal oblique increases IAP, providing the glottis is closed. Imagine the trunk as a cylinder. The top of the cylinder is formed by the diaphragm, the bottom the pelvic floor, and the walls the deep abdominals (transversus and internal oblique). As the abdominal wall is pulled in and up, the walls of the cylinder are effectively pulled in. If a deep breath is taken, the diaphragm is lowered, compressing the cylinder from the top. Providing the pelvic floor (the bottom of the cylinder) is intact, the cylinder is "pressurized" and made more solid. In this way, it is able to resist any bending stress applied to it.

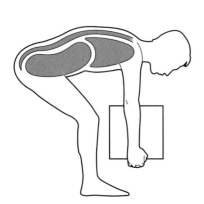

The IAP is greater if the breath is held following a deep inspiration (Valsalva maneuver) as the diaphragm is lower and the comparative size of the abdominal cavity (the cylinder) is reduced. During

Figure 3.15 Intra-abdominal pressure mechanism. Pressure within the abdomen acting against the pelvis and diaphragm provides additional extensor torque to the spine.

lifting, the pelvic floor muscles (the floor of the cylinder) contract to maintain pelvic integrity and prevent urination. The Valsalva maneuver is therefore appropriate in heavy lifting as long as it occurs only briefly. It must be borne in mind, however, that the blood pressure changes may not be desirable in subjects with poor cardiopulmonary health. Heavy lifting for this group is, therefore, not recommended.

Making the trunk into a more solid cylinder reduces axial compression and shear loads and transmits loads over a wider area (Twomey and Taylor 1987). IAP may also help to protect the spine from excessive indirect loads (those not acting directly on the spine but through limb loading), with the muscles acting to involuntarily fix the rib cage. IAP is greater when heavy lifts are performed and when the lift is rapid (Davis and Troup 1964).

Abdominal muscle strength affects IAP—strong athletes can produce very large IAP values (Harman et al. 1988). Yet strengthening the abdominal muscles with movements such as sit-ups does not permanently increase IAP (Hemborg et al. 1983) since these exercises usually do not mimic the coordination among abdominal muscles that is inherent in the IAP mechanism (Oliver and Middleditch 1991). Investigating the effect of abdominal muscle training on IAP, Hemborg et al. (1985) used isometric trunk curl and twist exercises. Increased recruitment of motor units in the oblique abdominal muscles clearly demonstrated muscle strengthening— yet EMG activity of these muscles decreased during lifting, implying that the subjects did not make functional use of their increased ability to recruit more motor units. The differentiation between increased strength and functional ability is an important one. If an exercise is not specific to a task being carried out, the physiological adaptation of the musculoskeletal system may be inappropriate. See page 99 for more discussion of training specificity.

KEY POINT: Sit-up exercises will not permanently raise intra-abdominal pressure.

A number of important criticisms has been made against the IAP mechanism when it has been presented as the *only* stabilizing process for the spine (Bogduk and Twomey 1987). First, to fully stabilize the spine during the lifting of heavy weights, the IAP would have to exceed the systolic pressure within the aorta, effectively cutting off the blood flow to the viscera and lower limbs. Competitive weight lifters have been known to black out when lifting extremely heavy weight, perhaps because of very high IAP (McGill et al. 1990). At the onset of a lift, there is an initial rapid rise in IAP—known as the snatch pressure—that may last for less than 0.5 second. The pressure declines during the remainder of the lift. Hemborg et al. (1985) calculated that a peak IAP of 250 mm Hg would be required to lift a 100-kg weight. Second, the muscle force required to create a sufficiently high IAP is greater than the hoop pressure possible from the abdominal muscles (Gracovetsky et al. 1985). Third, if the rectus abdominis contracts to increase IAP, it produces a flexion torque that counteracts the antiflexion effect of IAP created as the diaphragm and pelvic floor spread apart. These criticisms of IAP have led to reexamination of its contribution to back stability. Originally, IAP was believed to reduce the compression acting on the lumbar spine by as much as 40% (Eie 1966), but more recent studies have shown this to be only 7% (McGill et al. 1990).

KEY POINT: Intra-abdominal pressure has been estimated to reduce the compression acting on the lumbar spine by only 7%.

Bogduk and Twomey (1991) have considered a further effect of IAP in controlling axial rotation while lifting. Most mathematical models describe lifting in the sagittal plane only. From the functional standpoint, however, lifting is a multiplane activity, requiring stability to rotation as well as flexion-extension. If the internal and external obliques contract to control rotation, IAP may increase as a secondary effect.

SUMMARY

- The human spine is inherently unstable without its musculature.
- The interspinous and supraspinous ligaments, facet joint capsules, and thoracolumbar fascia (TLF) together provide passive support for the spine sufficient to balance between 24% and 55% of imposed flexion stress.
- The posterior ligamentous system stabilizes the spine passively and through elastic recoil.
- The TLF stabilizes the spine through three primary mechanisms: (1) passive resistance through its connections with the transversus abdominis muscle; (2) hydraulic amplification, as it restricts expansion of the erector spinae; and (3) "form closure" and "force closure" of the sacroiliac joint.
- Of the deep intersegmental muscles, the multifidus is most important for stabilizing the spine by helping to control lordosis and for neutralizing spinal flexion. Following lower-back injury, exercise therapy is required to restore multifidus function.
- Of the superficial back muscles, the erector spinae are most significant for back stabilization. It is their *endurance* rather than their strength that is particularly important.
- Of the abdominal muscles, the internal oblique and transversus abdominis are the major back stabilizers rather than the more

superficial external oblique and rectus abdominis. The *ratio* in which these muscles are used is more important that mere muscle strength.

- The key to effective abdominal training in sport is to train for trunk stability before training for trunk muscle performance.
- Individuals with low back pain tend to favor the more external abdominal muscles. Abdominal hollowing (rather than sit-ups), however, activates the internal oblique and transversus muscles—and since an important aim of rehabilitation is to help patients learn to dissociate use of the deeper muscles from use of the more superficial muscles, learning to practice abdominal hollowing is a vital part of rehabilitation.

II

Exercises for
Establishing Stability

Chapter 4 ("Teaching Your Clients the Basic Skills") is probably the most important chapter in this book. If you do no more than help your back pain clients to master all the movements in that chapter, you may well help them more than they would have been by a lifetime of standard weight training, exercises, massages, manipulations, etc.

But teaching your clients pelvic tilt, abdominal hollowing, how to assume the neutral lumbar position, and how to contract the multifidus (the essence of chapter 4) is just the beginning. The skills described in chapter 4 get your clients to the point where you can proceed with the rest of their treatment plans. You will want to identify and correct muscle imbalance as it is the source of much back pain and instability. Chapter 5 ("Muscle Imbalance") tells you how to diagnose imbalance and how to correct it. Chapter 6 ("Basic Abdominal Muscle Training") shows you how to teach your clients to train the abdominal muscles that most strongly affect low back pain—and these are *not* just the muscles that some therapists target when they assign "ab workouts" in order to deal with back problems. Your clients can do abdominal crunches until they have the most beautiful "six pack" on Malibu Beach and still be wracked with back pain. I show you how to target *all* the important structures (and they are not all muscles—you need to help your clients train their neurological responses as well!).

In chapter 7 ("Posture"), I show you how to determine if your clients have less-than-ideal posture and how to correct the different kinds of abnormal posture that can be a major factor in low back pain.

4

Teaching Your Clients the Basic Skills

Before your clients can follow rigorously the programs and practices discussed later in this book, they must have certain fundamental abilities. This chapter will help you understand how to teach your clients these skills.

Muscle action can stabilize the trunk effectively only if the trunk is a solid cylinder. In chapter 3, we saw that the deep (lateral) abdominal muscles (transversus abdominis and internal oblique) were the most important of the abdominal group for achieving this aim, whereas the multifidus is the most important of the back muscles. Our initial aim is to reeducate these muscles to gain voluntary control over their actions.

> **KEY POINT:** The back stability program begins with muscle reeducation. Before proceeding to the exercises described in later chapters, your clients should be able to control pelvic tilt; to identify and assume the neutral position of the lumbar spine; to perform abdominal hollowing; and to voluntarily contract the multifidus muscle.

Once your clients have achieved voluntary control, they are more able to use the muscles with minimal effort—the aim in all these exercises is for contraction intensities of only 30-40% of maximum, which can be easily sustained. Your clients must then learn to build the endurance of the muscles, aiming to perform 10 repetitions and hold each for 10 seconds. They also must learn to recognize the neutral position of the lumbar spine, to detect when the lumbar spine has moved away from this neutral position, and to correct the position of the lumbar spine using a pelvic tilting action.

TEACHING YOUR CLIENTS TO CONTROL PELVIC TILT

If you determine that your clients' lumbar-pelvic alignment is incorrect, you will need to teach them how to tilt and hold their pelvises in order to correct the misalignment. As you begin treatment, remember that for some, touching may be a sensitive issue. Be alert for words or body language that indicate tension in your client. Before you touch the client, explain clearly what you are going to do and be sure that she is comfortable with the proposed action. If not, try a different approach. With extra-sensitive clients, by proceeding gradually, you can usually establish the trust necessary to pursue the most helpful therapeutic course. Always bear in mind that therapist-client trust is an essential ingredient for successful treatment; do everything you can to establish and maintain that trust.

Segmental Control

The ability to dissociate the movement of one body segment from that of a neighboring segment is dependent on stabilization ability and adequate muscle length. The central requirement of segmental control as it applies to back stability is that the pelvis be able to tilt independently of the lumbar spine in both frontal and sagittal planes.

The combination of movements of the hip on the pelvis and of the lumbar spine on the pelvis increases the range of motion of this body area. The relationship between lumbar and pelvic movement is called **lumbar-pelvic rhythm** (see page 34). During forward flexion in standing, when the legs are straight, movement of the pelvis on the hip is limited to about 90° hip flexion. Any further movement, allowing the subject to touch the ground, must occur at the lumbar spine. For lumbar-pelvic rhythm to function correctly, movement of the pelvis on the hip should be equal to or greater than movement of the lumbar spine on the pelvis. In people with a history of back pain, however, the ability to perform pelvic tilting (pelvis moving on hip) is often lost—almost all the movement during forward bending comes from the lumbar spine, which shows excessive flexion laxity but limited, or often blocked, extension. In the lower trunk, the ability to *dissociate* lumbar movement from pelvic movement is therefore important, and correction of faulty lumbar-pelvic rhythm is vital.

> **KEY POINT:** The ability to dissociate movement of the lumbar spine from movement of the pelvis is essential for the healthy functioning of the back.

Assessing Lumbar-Pelvic Dissociation

You can use a variety of exercises to assess lumbar-pelvic rhythm; you may subsequently use the same exercises as part of the rehabilitation process. There is no stated "goal" for each of the following exercises because they all have basically the same goal: to allow you to assess your clients' abilities to dissociate lumbar from pelvic movement.

Knee Raising in Standing

The subject stands at a right angle to a wall bar for support, flexing his hip beyond 90° by raising his thigh to his chest and allowing his knee to bend. The movement should ideally occur in three phases. Initially there should be no pelvic or lumbar movement, with phase I consisting of hip flexion alone (a). During phase II, the pelvis should begin to posteriorly tilt as the hip approaches 90°. The lordosis should flatten, but the lumbar spine movement should not be excessive (b). In phase III, no further hip or pelvic movement is available, and the final position is obtained by lumbar flexion alone (c). When control of lumbar-pelvic rhythm is poor, lumbar flexion and pelvic rotation often occur early in phase I, with thoracic movement noticeable as the subject dips his chest downward toward the knee (d).

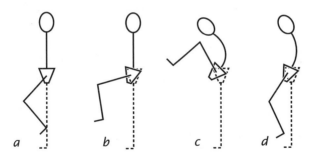

a　　　*b*　　　*c*　　　*d*

When lumbar flexion occurs early in the movement, the action of knee raising in standing can be used as a stability exercise in itself. Instruct your client to raise his knee initially by performing 10-20° hip flexion while maintaining stability of the lumbar-pelvic region and avoiding any pelvic tilt. To progress the overload of the exercise, increase the range of hip motion to 30-45° and slow the action so that the knee raise takes a total of 10 seconds.

Passive Assessment of Pelvic Tilt

While your client is standing, grip her below the waist with your forearm placed around the pelvic rim. Place your other hand flat on the sacrum, and use your shoulder to stabilize her thoracic spine. Move your client's pelvis into anterior and then into posterior tilt, assessing how far you can move it in either direction. If your client demonstrates a flatback posture, the amount of anterior tilt will be reduced; if she demonstrates a lordotic posture, the corresponding amount of posterior tilt will be limited.

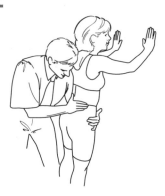

Assessing Lumbar-Pelvic Rhythm in Prone Kneeling

The subject sits back toward his ankles. Again, the action should occur in three phases. In phase I, no lumbar or pelvic movement should occur (a); in phase II, posterior pelvic tilt and hip flexion occur (b); and in phase III, lumbar flexion and some thoracic flexion finish the action (c). Faulty lumbar-pelvic rhythm often shows up immediately when lumbar flexion and posterior pelvic tilt occur immediately (d).

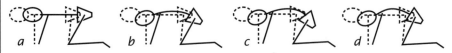

The Hip Hinge Movement in Standing

This activity permits you to observe your client's ability to isolate pelvic motion from that of the lumbar spine in the more functional position of standing. Your first aim is to assess the client's forward flexion since the relative contribution of anterior pelvic tilt to this movement is important. With normal lumbar-pelvic rhythm, unlocked knees and anterior pelvic tilt reduce the amount of lumbar flexion required to reach downward to below waist height, as when

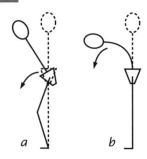

continued

The Hip Hinge Movement in Standing, continued

standing and working at a low bench (a). Where pelvic tilt is limited, greater lumbar flexion is required. Throughout the day, the number of lumbar flexion movements is greatly increased, leading to accumulated stress on the body tissues in this area (b).

Assessing Pelvic Motion Control in the Frontal Plane: The Trendelenburg Sign

When one leg supports all the body weight, the hip abductors (mainly gluteus medius) of the supporting leg work to prevent the pelvis from dipping (a). When these muscles are unable to hold an inner-range contraction, the pelvis dips downward toward the lifted leg, effec-

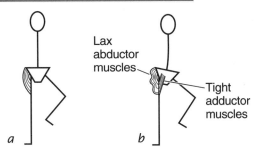

tively adducting the weightbearing limb (b). Persistent use of this action in the swayback posture can lead to an imbalance, combining lengthening of the hip abductors and shortening of the hip adductors.

Recognizing False Hip Abduction

In a nonweightbearing situation, inactivity of the gluteus medius shows as a false hip abduction movement. Normally when the upper leg is lifted from side lying, the pelvis remains level and the hip moves on this stable base (a). When the hip abductors are weak, the subject is unable to abduct the leg correctly (b).

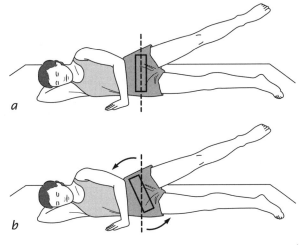

continued

Recognizing False Hip Abduction, continued

Instead, his pelvis tilts laterally on the spine using the trunk side flexors, which give the false appearance of hip abduction. Although the leg lifts, the relationship between the femur and pelvis remains unchanged, with close inspection showing the movement isolated to the lower spine.

Regaining Correct Lumbar-Pelvic Rhythm

The restoration of correct lumbar-pelvic rhythm is essential for the correct functioning of this region. Rehabilitation of this mechanism begins with your client recognizing the action of pelvic tilt and being able to maintain the neutral lumbar spine.

Control of lumbar-pelvic rhythm is used extensively during static loading of the stabilizing system covered in chapter 8 and during the rehabilitation of lifting in chapter 9. The following exercises will help your client gain the essential control of pelvic tilt that is necessary for basic back stability. The last two exercises use a gym ball and will prepare your client for the more advanced gym ball exercises described in chapter 9.

KEY POINT: The pelvic tilt mechanism is an important key to movements of the lumbar-pelvic region.

Assisted Pelvic Tilting While Standing

GOAL *For subjects who are unable to initiate a pelvic tilt.*

Promote passive movement while your clients are standing by gripping around their pelvic rim and supporting their sacrum with the flat of your opposite hand (as in "Passive Assessment of Pelvic Tilt," page 72). Push the pelvis into anterior tilt and then into posterior tilt, and have your clients attempt to return to the neutral position each time (i.e., to reproduce the passive motion) in order to enhance proprioceptive input to this area.

Assisted Pelvic Tilt While Sitting

GOAL *For subjects who are currently unable to perform a pelvic tilt while sitting. The action is especially useful for individuals whose flatback posture causes pain after prolonged sitting.*

Stand in front of your client and place a webbing belt around her waist. Gripping the belt, place your hand over her sternum to prevent upper body sway. As you pull the belt, her lumbar lordosis increases and her pelvis tends to tilt anteriorly. This action is made easier if your client sits on a wedge—in this case, the ischial tuberosities are higher than the pubic bone, and the pelvis is forced into anterior tilt.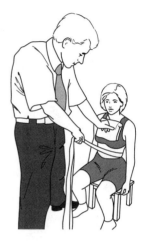

Initially, most of the power comes from your pulling on the belt, but gradually the belt provides less and less assistance as the subject becomes able to perform the tilting action by herself.

Assisted Pelvic Tilt From Crook Lying Position

GOAL *For subjects who are unable to perform a full active tilt by themselves in any position.*

The subject begins in the crook lying position, as for the heel slide maneuver on page 106. Grip his pelvis over the pelvic rim on each side, and push the pelvis into anterior and then posterior tilt. Encourage your subject to visualize the effect of the tilt on the lumbar spine as the lordosis is increased and reduced. Have him attempt first to follow the action using his own musculature (abdominals and gluteals), then gradually reduce your force in tilting the pelvis until he is performing the action independently.

Once your client can perform the action regularly in crook lying, he should attempt the same movements in the standing position. Begin with passive control (you provide the force for movement), then have your client gradually assume active control. Eventually have him perform pelvic tilting in a variety of starting positions including 4-point kneeling, 2-point kneeling, sitting, and supine lying. In each case the action of pelvic tilt is important, and the ability to reproduce the neutral lumbar position is essential. *continued*

Assisted Pelvic Tilt From Crook Lying Position, continued

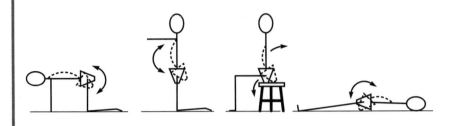

Hip Hinge Action in High (2-Point) Kneeling (Assisted)

GOAL *Uses a pelvic tilt action to move the spine forward and backward.*

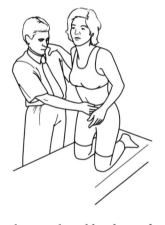

Once your subject can perform pelvic tilting well, she should combine it with classic "hip hinge" actions—where the trunk moves on the hip in a hinge action, and the spine remains straight. With your client in the 2-point kneeling position, assist her in performing the pelvic tilt. Encourage her to follow this movement with her shoulders, keeping her spine stable and avoiding any increase or decrease in lumbar lordosis. She should *gently* draw her abdominal muscles in (hollowing, see page 85) and maintain this minimal contraction (a feeling of "tightness" only) throughout the movement.

The essence of this action is to angle the spine forward and backward from the hip without flexing or extending the spine. The movement is made easier if the subject visualizes a rod tipping forward and backward from a single point (the hip) rather than a rope bending. You should provide gentle pressure on the back of your client's shoulders to initiate forward angulation of the spine and pressure over the front of the shoulder to initiate backward angulation. In each case, the spine remains straight, and the action comes from the spine (acting as a single unit) moving on the hip through pelvic tilting.

Hip Hinge (Table Support)

GOAL *A progression on assisted hip hinge.*

The subject stands facing a couch or other object placed just below waist level, with his hands on the couch surface (a). With his knees unlocked to relax the hamstring muscles, he performs the hip hinge action described in the previous exercise, using pelvic tilt and a fully stable spine. As he leans forward, he supports some of his weight with his hands, thus reducing spinal loading. After your client has mastered this supported action, he should move to the free standing position (b).

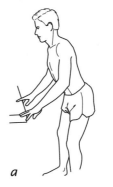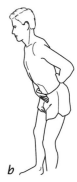

a   *b*

Controlled Forward Bending

GOAL *Teaches segmental control of the lumbar-pelvic region as a precursor to lifting.*

Once an individual has mastered the hip hinge actions, permit him a small degree of lumbar flexion—have him perform normal forward bend actions, with the pelvis initiating the action and both the pelvis and lumbar spine contributing equally throughout the first half of the range of motion.

Sitting Pelvic Tilt Using Gym Ball

GOAL *Teaches anterior-posterior pelvic tilt control.*

See chapter 9 for more thorough discussion of gym ball exercises and for more advanced exercises. The ball used is a standard 65-cm ball. Instruct your client to sit on the ball with her knees apart, feet flat on the floor. Both hips and knees should be flexed to about 90°. She should then tilt her pelvis alternately in both anterior and posterior directions, making sure that her shoulders and thoracic spine remain inactive. At first, she should attempt only small

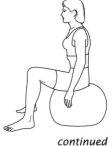

continued

Sitting Pelvic Tilt Using Gym Ball, continued

ranges of movement; as she gradually works up to larger ranges, the ball should roll forward and backward slightly.

Sitting Lateral Tilt Using Gym Ball

GOAL *Teaches lateral pelvic tilt control.*

Instruct your client to sit on the ball, as in the previous exercise, and to use lateral tilting to roll the ball from side to side, transferring the body weight from one ischial tuberosity to the other. Again, the shoulders should remain still throughout the action. The aim is to control the movement throughout the range using a smooth action and to avoid "falling into" the end-range position.

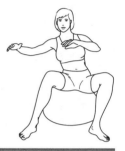

TEACHING YOUR CLIENTS TO IDENTIFY AND ASSUME THE NEUTRAL POSITION

Teaching clients to identify and maintain the neutral position of their lumbar spines is important for each stage of the back stability program since the neutral position places minimal stress on body tissues. **Lumbar neutral position** is midway between full flexion and full extension as brought about by posterior and anterior tilting of the pelvis. The discs and facet joints are minimally loaded in this position, and the soft tissues surrounding the lumbar spine are in elastic equilibrium. Because postural alignment is optimal in this position, it is generally the most effective position from which trunk muscles can work.

In the normal (nonpathological) person, the neutral position corresponds to lumbar alignment in an optimal posture. Individuals with suboptimal posture may increase or reduce their pelvic tilt, causing corresponding changes in the depth of lumbar lordosis. In either case, the neutral position remains midway between end-range flexion and end-range extension—in cases of postural malalignment, however, part of the treatment aim is to restore optimal posture by *rebalancing the length of the surrounding soft tissue elements*. Subjects can find neutral position passively (as you move the pelvis) or actively (subject moves her own pelvis through muscle action).

Refer to "Optimal Posture Alignment" in chapter 7 (page 134) for more thorough treatment of the neutral position while standing. In kneeling, your subject attempts similar lumbar alignment by slightly hollowing the lumbar spine. A flatback or excessive lordosis both mean that the subject has moved away from the neutral position and will need to reposition by tilting the pelvis.

With time, your clients will be able to recognize the neutral position and maintain it as appropriate. In the early stages of the program, however, you will need to constantly remind them of their spinal alignment. Proprioceptive exercises will help your client learn to assume neutral position at will.

Proprioception—Basic Concepts

Because proprioception is vital to the process of back stability during later stages of rehabilitation (Norris 1998), your clients should begin appropriate proprioceptive exercises at the start of their treatment programs. Lephart and Fu (1995) define **proprioception** as a specialized variation of touch encompassing the sensations of both joint movement and joint position. During acute injury, the reflexes initiated by displacement of mechanoreceptors and muscle spindles occurs far more rapidly than that brought about by pain (nociception) (Barrack and Skinner 1990). Effusion (escape of fluid) from joints contributes to a reduction in mechanoreceptor discharge, resulting in inhibition of muscular contraction. This inhibition commonly occurs in the vastus medialis (VMO) of the knee, for example, where just 60 ml of intra-articular effusion may result in 30-50% inhibition of quadriceps contraction (Kennedy et al. 1982). Proprioceptive deficits parallel joint degeneration (Barrett et al. 1991), but it is unclear whether this is a cause or a result of degeneration (Lephart and Fu 1995). Proprioceptive exercise is useful from the early stages of rehabilitation to restore normal functioning of the proprioceptive control of the back. And it is nowhere more useful than in helping your clients master assuming neutral position.

From a clinical standpoint, proprioception consists of three interrelating components (Beard et al. 1994) that represent activity at spinal, brain stem, and higher centers (Tyldesley and Grieve 1989) (table 4.1). Individuals

Table 4.1 Components of Proprioception

Level of neural system	Component of proprioception controlled
Spinal	Regulates muscle stiffness
Brain stem	Controls static joint positioning
Higher	Controls kinesthesia (movement sense)

beginning back stability training should focus on brain stem activities, characterized especially by static joint positioning, for they must cultivate this ability before proceeding to more advanced training.

Static Joint Positioning

Static joint position sense helps to maintain posture and balance at the brain stem level. Input for these actions is from joint proprioception, from the vestibular centers in the ears, and from the eyes. Balance and postural exercise with the eyes open or closed can enhance static joint position sense. Reproduction of passive positioning (RPP) and reproduction of active positioning (RAP) are exercises in which an individual tries to place a joint back in its starting position after either active or passive movement.

Reproduction of Passive Positioning

GOAL *To teach individuals how to maintain neutral position by improving the accuracy of body segment position.*

Four-point kneeling is the best starting position for restoring RPP during back stability training. Have your client kneel, with the lumbar spine in neutral position. After you passively move the spine away from neutral, instruct your client to place the spine back into the neutral position. Initially, you should work with single movements from flexion back to neutral and then extension back to neutral; then progress to combinations of movements—flexion-extension and lateral flexion and then back to neutral, for example. The aim is to increase the *precision* of movements so that the individual is able to accurately reproduce the neutral position alignment after each movement away from this starting position. After your client has mastered RPP in the 4-point kneeling position, move to other positions—especially those common to daily activities, such as sitting and standing.

Reproduction of Active Positioning

GOAL *To teach individuals how to maintain neutral position by improving the accuracy of movement.*

After your client has become proficient in passive positioning, he should initiate his own movements. Instruct him to begin in neutral position, move away from this position using single movements, and then move back into the neutral starting position. It sometimes works best if he

continued

Reproduction of Active Positioning, continued

begins RAP with a sitting or standing position—that way he can practice in front of a mirror, with his hands flat over his lower abdomen and sacrum to monitor pelvic tilt. Eventually, he uses no mirror and performs the movement without monitoring the action with his hands. Again, use a variety of movements from several starting positions.

KEY POINT: ▶ When performing exercises to improve reproduction of passive or active positioning (RPP/RAP), your client should focus on *precision* of movement.

TEACHING YOUR CLIENTS TO USE ABDOMINAL HOLLOWING

Individuals with low back pain must re-educate their muscles by learning to isolate the deep (lateral) abdominals from the superficial abdominals. This requires a hollowing action of the abdomen, using the internal oblique and transversus abdominis muscles (Lacote et al. 1987) rather than the traditional lumbar flexion movements (e.g., sit-ups) that emphasize the upper rectus (O'Sullivan et al. 1998). Before they can proceed with the exercises described later in this book, your clients must be able to perform abdominal hollowing well and consistently.

Because the concept of abdominal hollowing is probably less familiar than other major points in this chapter, I shall devote a disproportionately large portion of the chapter to this discussion.

Abdominal Hollowing—General Considerations

The **basic process of abdominal hollowing** is in theory simple and the same in all positions: the subject pulls the belly in and up at the navel without moving the rib cage, the pelvis, or the spine. Everything else in this section merely elaborates on that basic action and on how you can best help your clients to learn it well.

In comparison with mobilizer muscles (see page 92), stability muscles are better suited to endurance (postural holding) and better recruited at low resistance levels. Contraction intensities of 30-40% of the maximum voluntary contraction (MVC) work best for the deep (lateral) abdominal muscles. Your clients initially will have little control over the intensity of their contractions. Often they will begin with minimal contractions, then build to high intensities (60-70% MVC). This is acceptable during the early stages of learning and enables your clients to "feel the muscles working."

They eventually must gain accurate control, however, and you should instruct your clients to master changing the intensity of contraction in all hollowing exercises. An effective way to achieve this mastery is to ask for a maximal contraction, then tell your clients to relax by half, and then half again. Once they have achieved minimal contraction, they should then build up the intensity again, in steps, to the maximum. Only when they can control hollowing with minimal muscle intensity over a period of time (10 repetitions each of 30-40% MVC, held for 10 seconds) should they progress to more advanced exercises.

The position in which the movements are performed is important. Have your clients assume the *neutral position* of the spine whenever possible—initially, you will need to position your client correctly (you may want to read ahead to the section on "Optimal Postural Alignment" in chapter 7 [page 134] for the optimal position while standing). If your clients are kneeling, have them try to achieve proper alignment by slightly hollowing the lumbar spine—a flatback or excessive lordosis both mean that the subject has moved away from the neutral position and should appropriately reposition by tilting the pelvis. Eventually, your clients will be able to maintain the neutral position throughout their exercises.

KEY POINT: Have your clients maintain the neutral position of the spine throughout all the exercises in this chapter.

Abdominal Hollowing—Starting Positions

Different individuals require different starting positions, depending on their weight, degree of injury, flexibility, and so on. Standing (wall support) and 4-point kneeling are probably the easiest positions for most people.

Four-point kneeling places the fibers of the transversus abdominis muscle vertically. It thereby initiates some stretching in the transversus, making contraction of this muscle easier. The 4-point kneeling position is usually more comfortable than the other positions for people with back pain. On the other hand, 4-point kneeling requires control of structures in the spine, shoulders, and hips, whereas lying positions require control over only spinal structures. Since controlling a single body segment is considerably easier than controlling three, many people (especially those with poor body control, and especially when unsupervised) find exercises in the lying position easier to perform. Moreover, because 4-point kneeling places compression on the patellae and the wrists, individuals with pathology in these joints (such as arthritis) may need to modify the kneeling position. Modifications include (a) placing the open fist on the ground rather than the flat of the hand to reduce the wrist extension stress, (b) placing extra padding beneath the shins and leaving the patellae free,

(c) taking the body weight on the forearms rather than the wrists, and (d) supporting the upper body with the chest on a chair in order to reduce the upper body weight transmitted to the arms and wrists.

Obese subjects often have trouble performing abdominal hollowing in a kneeling position—the sheer weight of their abdominal tissue presents too large an overload for their deep abdominals to work against. For obese individuals, the standing (wall support) position is better: although it is usually a progression from kneeling (standing provides no stretch facilitation of the deep abdominals), obese individuals can control the action more easily. They can use their hands to palpate the abdominal wall, and the action of "pulling the tummy in" is often rather familiar in the standing position.

Prone lying is not suitable for obese individuals with poor abdominal muscle tone because of the compression of excess body tissue in this position. Lean people often like the prone position, however, since it provides many sensory cues—the act of hollowing to draw the abdominal wall away from the supporting surface gives useful tactile feedback (especially if a pressure biofeedback unit is used, as described later in this chapter).

You must use your own judgment to select appropriate starting positions for clients, taking into account body size, body condition, age, and pathology. Be flexible—experiment with different starting positions until your client feels comfortable with the exercise.

Abdominal Hollowing: 4-Point Kneeling

GOAL *To isolate the transversus abdominis and internal oblique.*

Because the transversus fibers are aligned horizontally, 4-point kneeling allows the abdominal muscles to sag, facilitating stretch. Position your client with her lumbar spine in a neutral position, her head looking at the floor, not forward, and her ears horizontally aligned to her shoulder joint. Her hip should be directly above the knee, her shoulder directly above the hand. The hands and knees are shoulder-width apart.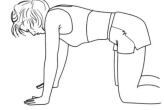

Instruct your client to focus her attention on her navel area, and to pull that region "in and up" while breathing normally. This action dissociates activity in the internal obliques and transversus from that of the rectus abdominis (Richardson et al. 1992). The exercise is thus useful for re-educating the stabilizing function of the abdominals when the rectus abdominis has become the dominant muscle of the group.

Abdominal Hollowing: Standing

GOAL *A progression from 4-point kneeling, or an initial position for obese individuals or others for whom 4-point kneeling is uncomfortable.*

Some subjects find 4-point kneeling difficult to control and tend to round their spines as they attempt abdominal hollowing. In this case, wall-supported standing is a more appropriate starting position. Your client should stand with his feet six inches from a wall and his back against the wall, while maintaining a neutral spinal position (a). An easy way to monitor neutral position is for your client to place one hand behind his back (over the sacrum) and the other in front of the abdomen, enabling him to monitor the position of his pelvis. He can also use his front hand to feel the contraction of the abdominal muscles as he initiates hollowing and draws the abdominal wall away from his hand.

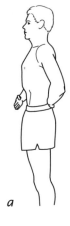

a

In an obese or poorly toned subject, the weight of the digestive organs will pull the abdominal wall out and down (visceral ptosis). If this occurs, position a belt below his navel (b), instructing him to contract the lateral abdominals and to pull the abdominal wall "in and up," trying to create a space between the abdomen and the belt.

Since motor programming links lateral abdominal action and pelvic floor action as part of the intra-abdominal pressure mechanism, pelvic floor contractions are also useful to aid learning of abdominal

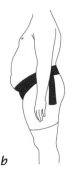

b

hollowing. Instruct your client to pull in the pelvic floor as though trying to stop himself from urinating. In men, the action of "lifting the penis" is also useful imagery.

KEY POINT: Linking abdominal hollowing with pelvic floor contractions is a useful way to enhance learning in both males and females.

It is important that your clients be able to differentiate the abdominal hollowing action from pelvic tilting. Be careful to ensure that your clients do not flatten their backs completely against the wall as that would indicate posterior pelvic tilting through action of the rectus abdominis. Once a client has performed wall-standing abdominal hollowing correctly to repetition, have him repeat the action without wall support. There should be no movement of the spine, pelvis, or rib cage.

Abdominal Hollowing: 2-Point Kneeling and Sitting

GOAL *For subjects who are already able to maintain the neutral lumbar position and control body sway.*

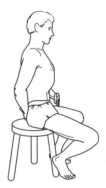

Two-point kneeling and sitting (stool) can help lead up to free standing, as they require greater body segment control than either lying or 4-point kneeling. This is because in both 2-point kneeling and sitting, the upper part of the trunk is unsupported, while in 4-point kneeling, the arms support the upper trunk. Individuals must be more active in controlling the upper trunk when it is unsupported, paying attention to the hollowing action as well as to the position of the lumbar spine (maintaining neutral position) and the position of their shoulders (avoiding body sway). These positions are also the starting points for the hip hinge actions described later. Have your clients pay close attention to movement of the rib cage, as well as to shoulder position, pelvic tilt, and maintenance of a neutral lordosis. Instructing your client to "sit tall" or "kneel tall" can facilitate correct alignment; this concept is also helpful in correcting whole-body posture while standing.

Abdominal Hollowing: Lying

GOAL *Suitable for lean individuals and those already able to perform hollowing.*

In *prone lying*, abdominal hollowing pulls the abdominal wall away from the floor—a practical cue for the beginning subject. Use of a pressure

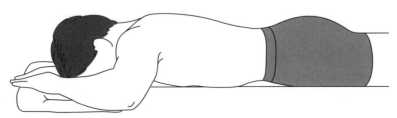

continued

Abdominal Hollowing: Lying, continued

biofeedback unit can be very helpful (consult a medical supply catalog). Note that the pressure biofeedback unit is useful only for assessment and not for continuing exercises. Place the bladder of the feedback unit below the navel, its lower edge in line with the anterior superior iliac spines. As your client performs hollowing, the dial of the biofeedback unit will show a decline in his body's pressure on the bladder. Once your client has mastered this action, you can link it with hip extension movements, if you wish, to provide abdominal-gluteal co-contraction.

Abdominal hollowing in *supine lying* permits an individual to feel the muscle activity and the pelvic position; again, pressure biofeedback may be useful. Have your client assume the crook lying position, with his fingers flat against the lateral abdominals below his navel. Explain that no pelvic tilt should occur during lateral abdominal contraction—you can check this by palpating the anterior superior iliac spine. You can use pressure biofeedback to monitor the depth of the lordosis: flattening of the back (posterior pelvic tilt) shows as increasing pressure on the dial and indicates activity of the rectus abdominis; excessive hollowing shows as reduced pressure and indicates loss of stability associated with anterior pelvic tilt.

As your client performs abdominal hollowing, the pressure biofeedback unit should register no more than a 5-mm Hg increase in pressure—at this level of pressure the internal oblique, the transversus abdominis, and the diaphragm are all recruited together. Higher values (up to 15 mm Hg) will not increase the recruitment of the deep abdominals but will increase the activity of both the diaphragm and the rectus abdominis (Allison et al. 1998).

Tips for Teaching Abdominal Hollowing

Multisensory cues can facilitate learning (Miller and Medeiros 1987). You can provide *auditory* cues by giving your clients frequent feedback about their performance; to create *visual* cues, encourage people to look at their muscles as they function and to place a mirror on the floor/couch below the abdomen; for *kinesthetic* cues, encourage subjects to "feel" the particular action—for example, ask them to "feel the stomach being pulled in."

KEY POINT: Multisensory cueing involves increased sensory input through auditory, visual, kinesthetic, and tactile stimuli, in conjunction with visualization of correct exercise technique.

Tactile cues for abdominal hollowing can come from you and/or from a belt touching your client's abdomen. The first technique involves **palpation.** Place the heel of your hand over the client's anterior superior iliac spine and point your fingers toward the pubic bone (figure 4.1). Your

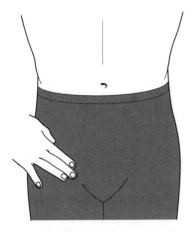

Figure 4.1 Palpation of the deep abdominals—the retroaponeurotic triangle—to teach abdominal hollowing.

fingertips will then fall over the retroaponeurotic triangle, which is the most superficial position of transversus abdominis (Walters and Partridge 1957). At this point the external oblique is aponeurotic and, so, not electrically active. This point may be used for siting the electrode of a surface EMG unit. Since the muscles are sheetlike, they will flatten rather than bulge when they contract. One way to facilitate the contraction is to instruct your clients to "stop me from pushing in" as you palpate the abdominal wall. A second way is have them cough (visceral compression) and hold the muscle contraction they feel beneath your fingers. This "cough and hold" procedure is also useful in conjunction with surface EMG—as the muscle contraction shows on the EMG unit, encourage the subject to maintain the contraction while breathing normally. Continue with this exercise until your client can hold the contraction for a single 30-second repetition or for 10 repetitions of 10 seconds each. Then encourage your client to *reduce* the contraction intensity of the muscle to the minimum required to maintain the hollow abdomen position.

Another tip for tactile cues in the 4-point kneeling position: fasten a **webbing belt** around your client's abdomen below the navel, with the muscles relaxed and sagging (figure 4.2). The belt should be just tight enough to touch the skin but not to pull in the muscles. Have your client hollow the abdomen, pull the muscles away from the belt, and then relax them completely to fill the belt again. Some people may be unable to draw the muscles away from the

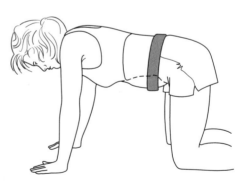

Figure 4.2 Using a belt to teach abdominal hollowing.

belt; others may contract their muscles too strongly, making the abdominal wall rigid and leading to an inability to relax the muscles again to fill the belt. Several days' practice will give your clients full muscle control over both actions. Once they can achieve the appropriate contraction, have them build up the holding time to 10-30 seconds while breathing normally.

A final learning technique is **visualization** of correct exercise technique following your demonstration. For this "mental practice," your clients should relax and "see" themselves performing the exercise in their imagination. Such visualization has been shown to benefit development of both motor skills (Fansler et al. 1985) and strength (Cornwall et al. 1991). To help your clients visualize the hollowing action, help them understand the workings of the transversus abdominis and internal oblique muscles—you can use simple diagrams of the muscles and then demonstrate their location using palpation. Analogies such as "personal muscle corset" or "cylinder of muscles" can be helpful.

Abdominal Hollowing: Common Errors

Be sure that your client's rib cage, shoulders, and pelvis remain still throughout the hollowing action (figure 4.3a). The contour of the abdomen will flatten if a person takes and holds a deep breath, but you will notice the chest expansion (figure 4.3b). If this occurs, instruct your client to exhale and then hold the resulting chest position while performing the exercise. Placing a belt around the lower chest provides helpful feedback about chest movement (Richardson and Hodges 1996). If your client is using the external oblique to brace the abdomen, which is also an incorrect technique, the lower ribs will be depressed, and you may observe a horizontal skin crease across the upper abdomen (figure 4.3c). When this occurs, instruct your client to perform pelvic floor contraction at the same time as abdominal hollowing, but to *avoid* contracting the gluteus maximus (use of which leads in this case to inappropriate motor patterns for trunk stability during dynamic sports activity).

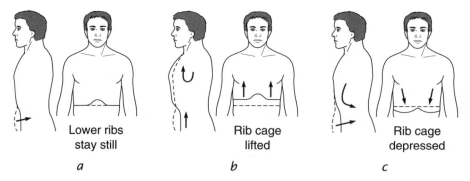

Lower ribs stay still

a

Rib cage lifted

b

Rib cage depressed

c

Figure 4.3 Abdominal hollowing in standing: *(a)* is correct, and *(b)* and *(c)* are incorrect.

In kneeling, lying, and sitting positions, pressing onto the floor with the feet indicates a failure to isolate the deep abdominal action from that of the hip muscles. Placing your client's feet on a bathroom scale will provide clear feedback about hip extension pressure—ideally, the scales should show no increase in weight during the exercise.

KEY POINT: Your clients should maintain a neutral lumbar position during abdominal hollowing and refrain from significant movement of ribs, pelvis, or hips.

TEACHING YOUR CLIENTS TO CONTRACT THE MULTIFIDUS MUSCLES AT WILL

Multifidus is the key stabilizer muscle within the spinal extensor group (page 50). Subjects with low back pain often lose the ability to contract this muscle (probably through pain inhibition), and they do not regain the ability spontaneously (Hides et al. 1996). Two kinds of exercises will help increase your client's basic back stability. The first focuses solely on the multifidus muscles, with an emphasis on helping your client learn to recognize what it feels like to tension/relax *only* those particular muscles. The second, using the techniques of proprioception, focuses not only on the multifidus but also on the lateral abdominals, which of course are also vital for basic stability.

The Basic Exercise for Multifidus Contraction

Your help is essential for your client to learn adequate control of this muscle.

Multifidus Contraction

GOAL *To learn to use the multifidus at will and separately from other muscles.*

Your client begins in a prone lying position while you palpate his lower back medial to the longissimus at L4 and L5 levels. Identify the spinous processes and slide your fingers laterally into the hollow between the spinous process and the longissimus bulk. Assess the difference in muscle consistency, and then determine your client's ability to isometrically contract the multifidus in a "setting" action. Once the individual can consciously contract the muscle, encourage him to use multifidus setting

continued

Multifidus Contraction, continued

in a sitting position with a neutral lumbar spine. He should become able to symmetrically contract the two multifidus muscles and sustain the contraction for 10-30 seconds.

Rhythmic Stabilization

Rhythmic stabilization involves gross action of the multifidus in conjunction with the lateral abdominals. **Rhythmic stabilization** is a PNF (proprioceptive neuromuscular facilitation) technique that involves alternating isometric contractions of the agonist and antagonist muscles, building up to co-contraction (Sullivan et al. 1982). The general idea is simple: first, you apply a resistance in one direction and your client contracts her muscle against the resistance. Once you feel that the contraction has reached a maximum, instantaneously apply your resistance in the opposite direction—at which point she contracts the antagonist muscle, with *no momentary relaxation* between the two contractions. In this way, the muscle pairs are contracting to gradually higher levels. The following exercise uses this technique in teaching your client to contract the multifidus.

Rhythmic Stabilization of Multifidus and Lateral Abdominals in Side Lying Position

GOAL *To encourage your client to contract the multifidus and lateral abdominals simultaneously.*

With your client in the crook side lying position, palpate the intervertebral joints to ascertain the midpoint of the movement range at the spinal level where you have found pain/pathology (Maitland 1986). Remember that the multifidus muscle is unisegmental—that is, each fascicle stretches over only a single segment of the lumbar spine. Wasting of the muscle occurs at the same level as the segment of pathology (Hides et al. 1994). To place the relevant muscle fascicle at its optimum length, you must move the painful segment into its midrange. *If you feel inadequate to do this, ask an experienced orthopedic physical therapist to work with you.*

The exercise consists of you pushing forward on your client's pelvis and backward onto the shoulder while your client resists the action. Then reverse the action: while you push backward on the pelvis and forward onto the shoulder, she continues to resist the action, not allowing herself to relax even for a second. The action can be more localized by an orthopedic physical therapist who can palpate the specific spinal

continued

> *Rhythmic Stabilization of Multifidus and Lateral Abdominals in Side Lying Position, continued*
>
> level that requires resistance to rotation. General resisted rotation can be performed for the whole spine by having a partner help you use this exercise at home.
>
> The exercise is repeated 5-10 times at each of three treatment sessions.

Teaching Tips for Multifidus Contraction

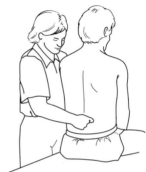

Figure 4.4 Palpating to assist your client in detecting multifidus contraction.

From Norris 1998.

Initially, you will palpate with your thumb and the knuckle of your first finger placed on either side of the lumbar spinous process at any one level. Instruct your client to "feel the muscle swelling" without actively flexing the lumbar spine (figure 4.4). You may want to suggest that your client practice this action with his own thumbs so he'll have some feedback for home practice. While sitting, he should press into the extensor region with his thumbs at the side of the spinous processes. The pressure should be steady but deep. The aim is to feel the muscle swelling against his digital pressure without allowing his pelvis to tilt or his spine to arch. Angling the trunk forward at the hip (hip hinge action) will contract the longissimus and enable your client to distinguish between the longissimus fibers (more lateral) and the multifidus. Performing abdominal hollowing at the same time will improve the multifidus contraction.

SUMMARY

- Safely improving back stability requires that an individual learn to contract certain muscles voluntarily and independently—in particular, the deep abdominal muscles (transversus abdominis and internal oblique) and the multifidus muscles of the back.
- Such independent muscle control enables an individual
  1. to control pelvic tilt (i.e., to voluntarily move the pelvis independently of the spine);
  2. to support the spine with contracted multifidus;
  3. to support the spine with abdominal hollowing; and
  4. to achieve the neutral position of the lumbar spine, from which position most exercises in this book should begin.
- This chapter teaches you, the therapist, how to help your clients learn these skills.

5
Muscle Imbalance

Muscle imbalance occurs when a particular agonist is significantly stronger than its antagonist, or when one or the other is abnormally shortened or stretched. The body's attempts to compensate for imbalance generally exacerbate the problem and can lead to serious disability. This chapter first presents general theory about muscle balance and imbalance. It then shows you how to identify such problems and how to treat them. Much of the material for this section is modified from Norris (1998), to which you are referred for further reading.

BASIC CONCEPTS

We can categorize muscles into two nondistinct groups (Janda and Schmid 1980; Richardson 1992): (1) Muscles that primarily stabilize a joint and approximate the joint surfaces are known as **stabilizers** or "postural muscles." (2) Muscles primarily responsible for movement (those which develop angular rotation more effectively than the stabilizers), are called **mobilizers** or "task muscles."

> **Terms You Should Know**
>
> **diastasis** separation of normally joined parts.
> **pseudoparesis** apparent weakness brought on by increased tone in a muscle antagonist.

KEY POINT: Stabilizers (postural muscles) primarily fix a joint and prevent movement. Mobilizers (task muscles) primarily create movement.

Stability muscles tend to be more deeply placed in the body and are usually monoarticular (one-joint) muscles, whereas mobilizers are on the whole superficial and are often biarticular (two-joint) muscles. For example, in the leg, the rectus femoris is classified as a mobilizer, while the other

---

Chapter 5 exercise descriptions adapted from Norris 1998.

quadriceps muscles are stabilizers. Stabilizer function is more slow-twitch (type I) or tonic in nature, whereas that of the mobilizers tends toward fast-twitch (type II) action. This physiology suits the functional requirements of the muscles—enabling mobilizers to contract and develop maximal tension rapidly but also to fatigue quickly. The stabilizer muscles build tension slowly and perform well at lower tensions over longer periods, being more fatigue-resistant.

Stabilizers can be subdivided into primary and secondary types (Jull 1994) (table 5.1). The primary stabilizers (e.g., multifidus, transversus abdominis, and vastus medialis oblique) have very deep attachments, lying close to the axis of rotation of the joint. In this position, they are unable to contribute any significant torque but will approximate the joint.

Table 5.1 Muscle Types

The following characteristics are not absolute but are only tendencies within these sometimes inexact categories of muscles.

Stabilizers		Mobilizers
▪ Primarily responsible for stabilizing and approximating joints		▪ Primarily responsible for movement, including angular rotation
▪ Examples: multifidus, transversus abdominis, vastus medialis oblique		▪ Examples: rectus femoris, hamstrings
Primary stabilizers	**Secondary stabilizers**	
▪ Deep, close to joint	▪ Intermediate depth	▪ Superficial
▪ Slow twitch	▪ Slow twitch	▪ Fast twitch
▪ Usually monoarticular (1 joint)	▪ Usually monoarticular	▪ Often biarticular (2 joints)
▪ No significant torque	▪ Primary source of torque	▪ Secondary source of torque
▪ Short fibers	ments multipinnate	
▪ Build tension slowly, more fatigue resistant		▪ Build tension rapidly, fatigue quickly
▪ Better activated at low levels of resistance		▪ Better activated at high levels of resistance
▪ More effective in closed chain movement		▪ More effective in open chain movements
▪ In muscle imbalance, tend to weaken and lengthen		▪ In muscle imbalance, tend to tighten and shorten

In addition, many of these smaller muscles have important propriocep-tive functions (Bastide et al. 1989). The secondary stabilizers (e.g., gluteals and oblique abdominals) are the main torque producers, being large monoarticular muscles attaching via extensive aponeurosis. Their multipinnate fiber arrangement makes them powerful and able to ab-sorb large amounts of force through eccentric action. The mobilizers (e.g., rectus femoris and hamstrings) act as stabilizers only in conditions of extreme need. They are fusiform in shape—a less powerful fiber arrange-ment, but one able to produce large ranges of motion.

Stabilizer muscles are better activated at low resistance levels—about 30-40% of the maximum voluntary contraction (MVC)—while mobilizer muscles are generally better activated above this level. Re-educating the muscles of back stability therefore calls for low-level contractions, *not* the extreme workouts well-meaning therapists sometimes prescribe for lower back pain. In addition, stabilizer muscles respond better to closed kinetic chain actions, where movement occurs proximally on a stabilized distal segment; in standing, this would be with the foot on the ground for the lower limb, or the hand on a wall for the upper limb. Mobilizer function is more effective in an open chain situation, where free movement occurs without distal fixation. In the lower limb, the swing phase of gait is open chain; in the upper limb, throwing is a prime example. The structure and functional characteristics of the two muscle categories makes the stabiliz-ers better equipped for postural holding and antigravity function. The mobilizers are better designed for rapid ballistic movements.

Two fundamental changes appear when there is muscle imbalance: (1) **tightening** of mobilizer (two-joint) muscles and (2) loss of endurance (**holding**) within the inner range of motion of the (single-joint) stabilizer muscles, which arises from their being abnormally stretched. These two changes are used as tests for the degree of muscle imbalance present. Since the changes in length and tension alter muscle pull around a joint, they may draw the joint out of alignment. Changes in body segment alignment and the degree of **segmental control** (the ability to move one body seg-ment without moving any others) form the basis of the third type of test used when assessing muscle imbalance. The mixture of tightness and weak-ness in muscle imbalance alters body segment alignment and changes the equilibrium point of a joint. Normally, the equal resting tone of agonist and antagonist muscles allows the joint to assume a balanced resting po-sition, with the joint surfaces evenly loaded and the joint's inert tissues not excessively stressed. However, if the muscles on one side of a joint are tight and the opposing muscles are lax, the joint will be pulled out of align-ment toward the tight muscle (figure 5.1). This alteration in alignment throws weightbearing stress onto a smaller region of the joint surface, in-creasing pressure per unit area. Further, the inert tissues on the shortened (closed) side of the joint will contract over time.

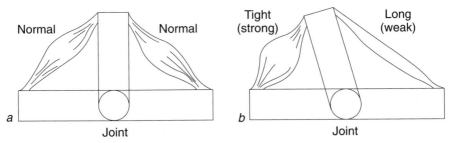

Figure 5.1 Posture and muscle imbalance. *(a)* Equal muscle tone gives correct joint alignment. *(b)* Unequal muscle tone pulls joint out of alignment, resulting in faulty posture.

Reprinted from Griffin 1998.

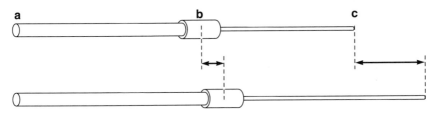

Figure 5.2 Relative flexibility. When the attached cords are stretched, the tighter cord (A–B) moves less than the looser cord (B–C).

From Norris 1998.

Imbalance also leads to a lack of accurate segmental control. The combination of stiffness (hypoflexibility) in one body segment and laxity (hyperflexibility) in an adjacent segment leads to relative flexibility (White and Sahrmann 1994). In a chain of movement, the body seems to take the path of least resistance, with the more flexible segment always contributing more to the total movement range. Consider two pieces of rubber tubing of unequal strengths that are attached to one another (figure 5.2). If the movement begins at C and A is fixed, the more flexible area B-C moves more. This will still be the case if C is held immobile and A moves.

Taking this example into the body, figure 5.3 shows a toe-touching exercise. The two areas of interest for relative flexibility are the

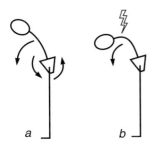

Figure 5.3 Relative stiffness in the body. *(a)* Forward flexion should combine equal pelvic tilt and spinal flexion. *(b)* Tight hamstrings limit pelvic tilt, stressing the more lax spinal tissues.

(a) From Norris 1998.

hamstrings and lumbar spine tissues. As we flex forward, movement should occur through a *combination* of anterior pelvic tilt and lumbar spinal flexion. Many people have tight hamstrings and excessively lax lumbar tissues due to excessive bending (lumbar flexion) during everyday activities. During this flexing action, greater movement (and therefore greater tissue strain) always occurs at the lumbar spine. *Relative stiffness in this case makes the toe-touching exercise ineffective as a hamstring stretch unless the trunk muscles are tightened to stabilize the lumbar spine.*

> **KEY POINT:** Muscle imbalance can lead to changes in both function and structure of the body tissues.

MUSCLE ADAPTATION TO INJURY, IMMOBILIZATION, AND TRAINING

Different kinds of muscles react differently to injury and immobilization. Primary stabilizers such as multifidus and transversus abdominis, for example, react quickly (by inhibition) to pain and swelling (see table 5.2).

Table 5.2 Stabilizer and Mobilizer Muscles That Affect the Lower Back

Muscles marked with * can act as both stabilizers and mobilizers, in different situations.

Stabilizers	Mobilizers

• Primary stabilizers
  Multifidus
  Transversus abdominis
  Internal oblique
  Gluteus medius
  Vastus medialis
  Serratus anterior
  Lower trapezius
  Deep neck flexors
	• Iliopsoas*
	• Hamstrings
	• Rectus femoris
	• Tensor fasciae lata (TFL)
	• Hip adductors
	• Piriformis
	• Rectus abdominis

• Secondary stabilizers
  Gluteus maximus
  Quadriceps
  Iliopsoas*
  Subscapularis
  Infraspinatus
  Upper trapezius*
  Quadratus lumborum*
	• External oblique
	• Quadratus lumborum*
	• Erector spinae
	• Sternomastoid
	• Upper trapezius*
	• Levator scapulae
	• Rhomboids
	• Pectoralis minor
	• Pectoralis major
	• Scalenes

There are even more clear differences in reactions to reduced usage, which has been studied extensively using immobilized limbs. The greatest tissue changes occur within the first few days of disuse. Strength loss can be as much as 6% per day for the first eight days, with minimal loss after this period (Appell 1990).

Type I and type II muscle fibers differ considerably in response to disuse, with type I fibers showing greater reduction in size and greater loss of total fiber numbers than type II. In fact, the number of type II fibers actually increases—demonstrating a process of selective atrophy of the type I fibers (Templeton et al. 1984). However, not all muscles show an equal amount of type I fiber atrophy. Atrophy is largely related to change in use relative to normal function, with the initial percentage of type I fibers that a muscle contains being a good indicator of likely atrophy pattern. Those muscles with a predominantly antigravity function, which cross one joint and have a large proportion of type I fibers (e.g., the soleus and vastus medialis muscles) show greatest selective atrophy. Predominantly slow twitch antigravity muscles that cross multiple joints are next in order of atrophy (e.g., erector spinae). Finally, the phasic, predominantly fast type II muscles (e.g., biceps) can be immobilized with less loss of strength than the other two groups (Lieber 1992).

Training also causes selective changes in muscle. In the knee, rapid flexion-extension actions can selectively increase activity in the rectus femoris and hamstrings (biarticular mobilizers) but not in the vasti (monoarticular stabilizers). In a study by Richardson and Bullock (1986) comparing speeds of 75°/sec and 195°/sec, mean muscle activity for the rectus femoris increased from 23.0 μV to 69.9 μV. In contrast, muscle activity for the vastus medialis increased from 35.5 μV to only 42.3 μV (figure 5.4). The pattern of muscle activity was also noticeably different after training. The rectus femoris and hamstrings displayed phasic (on-and-off) activity at the fastest speeds, while the vastus medialis showed a tonic (continuous) pattern. The graphs in figure 5.5 show an EMG trace of the electrical activity produced when a muscle contracts. The general trend of the graph *shape* is important, rather than each individual line. Note that there are clear groups of electrical spikes for the rectus femoris and the hamstrings, indicating that activity occurred in these muscles at specific points in the total movement. For the vastus medialis there are no clear groups, indicating that the activity occurred continually throughout the movement.

Ng and Richardson (1990) found similar changes even in the more functional closed kinetic chain position. A four-week training period of rapid plantar flexion (in standing position) gave significant increases in jump height (gastrocnemius, biarticular) but also significant losses of static function of the soleus (monoarticular).

Recruitment patterns of lower back muscles also change depending on the type of training used (O'Sullivan et al. 1998). Subjects followed a

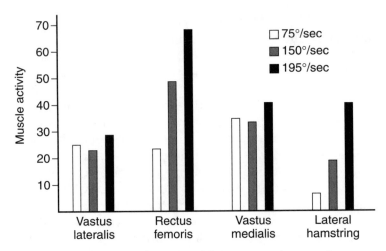

Figure 5.4 Muscle activity changes with increases in speed.
Reprinted from Richardson and Bullock 1986.

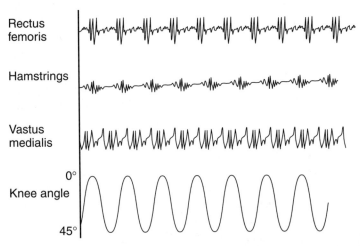

Figure 5.5 Muscle activity patterns during rapid alternating knee flexion-extension. Note that biarticular muscles are phasic, while monoarticular muscles are tonic.

Reprinted from Richardson and Bullock 1986.

10-week training program involving either abdominal hollowing (15 minutes daily, progressed with limb loading) or gym exercise that included trunk curls. EMG activity of the internal oblique (more important for back stability) increased in the hollowing group, whereas that of the rectus abdominis remained relatively unchanged. Trunk curls (but

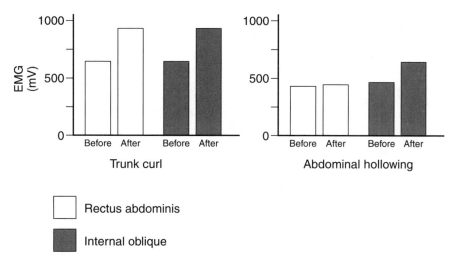

Figure 5.6 Altered abdominal muscle recruitment pattern with training.
Data from O'Sullivan et al. 1998.

not hollowing) led to an increase in rectus abdominis activity and a reduction in activity of the internal oblique (figure 5.6).

TRAINING SPECIFICITY

The aforementioned differences in responses of stabilizer and mobilizer
muscles illustrate the importance of training specificity. Responses to training closely correspond to the type of exercise used. For example, if runners want to reduce their marathon running time, sprint training will not
be effective. This is because sprinting is primarily an anaerobic activity
(energy supplied from stores within the body), whereas marathon training is predominantly aerobic (energy supplied by using oxygen and food
as fuel). We can say in this case that, although the sprint training caused
an increase in fitness, the aspect of fitness that improved was not strictly
relevant to the event that the training was designed for. The training was
not *specific* to the event.

In the same way, we have seen that high-speed muscle training leads to
recruitment of mobilizer muscles. In the example from Richardson and
Bullock (1986) described previously, the rectus femoris increased its activity markedly at high-speed (195°/sec) movements. If we used this high-
speed training to try to improve the vastus medialis, it would not be very
effective.

Specificity can be remembered by a simple mnemonic, **S.A.I.D.,** which
stands for **S**pecific **A**daptation to **I**mposed **D**emand. The change occurring in the body (the adaptation) is specific to (exactly matches) the training used (the imposed demand). You can adequately address your clients'

muscle imbalances only by using quite specific exercises—which, of course, require equally *accurate, specific assessments* of which muscles need what kind of treatment. The tests described later in this chapter will help you make such appropriate assessments.

> **KEY POINT:** Training specificity dictates that, when designing an exercise program for a client, you must consider the functional requirements, contraction type, and speed of contraction of a muscle.

CHANGES IN MUSCLE LENGTH

Changes in muscle length do not occur in a uniform manner throughout the body. An overly simplistic but useful description is that stabilizer muscles tend to "weaken" (sag), whereas mobilizers tend to "shorten" (tighten). Exercise therapy aimed at muscle must therefore be selective rather than general, seeking to lengthen (stretch) tight mobilizer muscles and shorten/build endurance of inactive stabilizer muscles.

Chronic Muscle Lengthening

The weakening of stabilizer muscles has been termed **stretch weakness** (Kendall et al. 1993): the muscle remains in an elongated position, beyond its normal resting position but *within* its normal range. This is different from **overstretch,** in which the muscle is elongated *beyond* its normal range.

The length-tension relationship of a muscle (page 38) dictates that a stretched muscle, where the actin and myosin filaments are pulled apart, can exert less force than a muscle at normal resting length. Where the stretch is maintained, however, this short-term response (reduced force output) becomes a long-term adaptation: the muscle adds more sarcomeres to its ends in an attempt to move its actin and myosin filaments closer together (figure 5.7). This adaptation, known as an increase in **serial sarcomere number (SSN),** can lengthen a muscle by up to 20% (Gossman et al. 1982).

The length-tension curve of an adaptively lengthened muscle moves to the right (figure 5.8). The peak tension such a muscle can produce in the laboratory is up to 35% greater than that of a normal length muscle (Williams and Goldspink 1978). However, this peak tension occurs at approximately the position where the muscle has been immobilized (point a, figure 5.8). If the strength of the lengthened muscle is tested with the joint in midrange or inner range (point b, figure 5.8), as is common in clinical practice, the muscle cannot produce its peak tension and appears "weak." For this reason, manual muscle tests appear to be more accurate indicators of positional strength than measures of total strength (Sahrmann 1987).

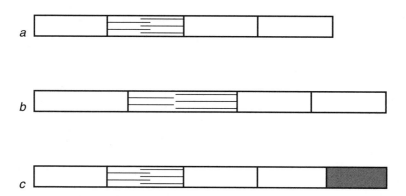

Figure 5.7 Muscle length adaptation. *(a)* Normal muscle length. *(b)* In stretched muscle, the filaments move apart, resulting in loss of muscle tension. *(c)* Normal filament alignment is restored by increases in serial sarcomere number (SSN), resulting in chronic abnormal muscle length.

From Norris 1998.

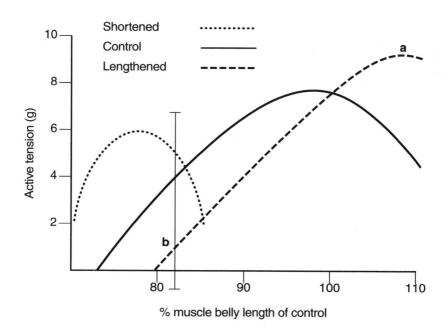

Figure 5.8 Effects of immobilizing a muscle in shortened and lengthened positions (see text for explanation).

From Norris 1998.

In the laboratory, a lengthened muscle returns to its optimal length within approximately one week if placed in a shortened position (Goldspink 1992). Clinically, restoration of optimal length may be achieved by immobilizing the muscle in its physiological rest position (Kendall et al. 1993) and/or by exercising it in its shortened (inner-range) position (Sahrmann 1990). *Enhancement of strength is* not *the priority in this situation*—indeed, the load on the muscle may need to be reduced to ensure correct alignment of the various body segments and correct performance of the relevant movement pattern.

SSN may be partly responsible for changes in muscle strength without parallel changes in hypertrophy (Koh 1995). A number of factors influence SSN, which exhibits marked plasticity. For example, immobilization of rabbit plantarflexors in a lengthened position showed an 8% increase in SSN in only four days; applying electrical stimulation to increase muscle force led to an even greater increase (Williams et al. 1986). Stretching a muscle appears to affect SSN significantly more than does immobilization in a shortened position. Following immobilization in a shortened position for two weeks, the mouse soleus decreased SSN by almost 20% (Williams 1990). However, stretching for just one hour per day in this study not only eliminated the SSN reduction, but actually increased SSN by nearly 10%. Eccentric stimuli appear to cause a greater adaptation of SSN than concentric stimuli. Morgan and Lynn (1994) subjected rats to uphill or downhill running and found SSN in the vastus intermedius to be 12% greater in the eccentric-trained rats after one week. Koh (1995) has suggested that, if SSN adaptation occurs in humans, strength training may produce such a change if it is performed at a joint angle different from that at which the maximal force is produced during normal activity.

The lengthened muscle is not weak—it merely lacks the ability to maintain full contraction within the inner range. This shows up clinically as a difference between the active and passive inner ranges. If the joint is passively placed in full anatomical inner range, the subject is unable to hold the position. Sometimes the position cannot be held at all, but more usually the contraction cannot be sustained, indicating a lack in slow twitch endurance capacity.

Clinically, reduction of muscle length is seen as the enhanced ability to hold an inner-range contraction. This may or may not represent a reduction in SSN but is a required functional improvement in postural control for muscles that are abnormally lengthened. Muscle shortening appears in the dorsiflexors of equestrians, who clearly do not hold the shortened position permanently, as with splinting, but rather show a training response. Following pregnancy, SSN increases in the rectus abdominis in combination with diastasis. Again, length of the muscle gradually reduces in the months following birth. Inner-range training, then, is likely to shorten a lengthened muscle (Goldspink 1996).

Assessing Stretched Muscles— Testing Inner-Range Holding Ability

We have seen from figure 5.8 that the length-tension curve of a lengthened muscle moves to the right, indicating that it is unable to produce significant power within the full inner range. This fact forms the basis of the assessment of stabilizer muscle length by inner-range holding tests. Tests for the most important stabilizing muscles are described below.

Lower Back and Hip Muscles—Inner-Range Holding Tests

The ability of a stabilizer to maintain a low-load isometric contraction over a period of time is vital to its antigravity function and may be assessed using the standard muscle test position (Richardson 1992; Richardson and Sims 1991). In all the following assessments, ask your clients to maintain a contraction in full inner range, the key factor being the length of time they can maintain the static hold before developing jerky (phasic) movements. In each case, you will place the limb passively into the full inner range. If the limb drops upon release, the passive range of motion differs from the active range—an important indicator of poor stabilizer function. Full stabilizing function is present only when a subject can maintain the inner-range position for 10 repetitions of 10 seconds' duration (Jull 1994). In all the tests, it is important that your subjects attempt all 10 repetitions; often they will perform the first two or three normally, with the deficit becoming apparent only in later repetitions.

Assessing Muscle Balance in the Iliopsoas

While sitting, your client flexes her hip while maintaining 90° knee flexion so that the foot is lifted clear of the ground. Have her hold this position as long as she can, while you record the time at which phasic movements begin. Note also the position of the pelvis and lumbar spine. Where the iliopsoas is lengthened, one of two things may happen: (1) If lumbar stability is poor, the pelvis will drop back into posterior tilt, flattening or even reversing the lumbar lordosis. (2) If lumbar stability is good, your client will be able to maintain the neutral position of the lumbar spine and pelvis—but the knee will simply drop, indicating that the hip flexor muscles have lengthened (but not necessarily weakened) and are unable to hold the full inner-range position.

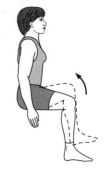

Assessing Muscle Balance in the Gluteus Maximus

Have your client lie in a prone position with her knee flexed to 90°. Then she should lift her hip to the inner range of extension and hold it steady (right; b, below). Using palpation, note the order of muscle 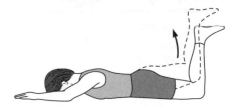 contraction during the hip extension. Normally, the hamstrings should contract first, followed by the gluteus maximus, then the contralateral erector spinae, and finally the ipsilateral erector spinae (Lewit 1991). In many cases of imbalance, the gluteus is poorly recruited or even inhibited (pseudoparesis) by tightness in the opposing hip flexors (Janda 1986). Where this is the case, the order of muscle contraction changes. If the gluteals do not function adequately, the hamstrings dominate the movement—little gluteal activity is apparent, and the muscle mass remains flaccid. Note how long your client can hold the position steady before phasic movement begins.

Performing the test with the knee bent reduces the contribution that the hamstrings make to the movement by shortening them. The contribution of the gluteus is therefore more apparent. Your ability to see and feel the subtle changes that indicate the order of muscle contraction, however, takes time to develop. Until you have gained experience in this area of examination, you can use dual-channel EMG to show the intensity and timing of muscle contraction. Note: watch carefully to see if your client performs a false hip extension movement; in this action, the pelvis anteriorly tilts due to powerful action of the erector spinae, and the relationship between the hip and pelvis remains the same (c).

Thoroughly explain to your client which muscles she should be using to perform this activity and in which order. If she tends to make a false hip extension, hold her pelvis down while she raises her leg using only her gluteals, so that that she learns what the correct movement feels like.

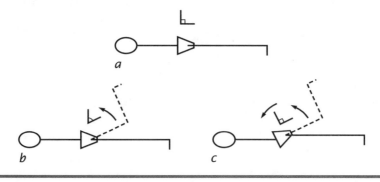

Assessing Muscle Balance in the Gluteus Medius

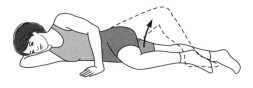

The action in this test is combined hip abduction, with slight lateral rotation to emphasize the posterior fibers of the muscle. Have your client lie on her side with her upper knee flexed. Instruct her to abduct and externally rotate her upper leg so that the femur is at a 45° angle to the ground and her knee is flexed about 45° (dotted lines in figure). Then have her rotate her chest toward the examination table while keeping her upper leg in place (Jull 1994).

Deep Abdominal Muscles—Inner-Range Holding Tests

Rather than deal with specific abdominal muscles as I did with the hip muscles, I think it more useful in this section to focus on the entire system of deep abdominal muscles that affect lumbar stability and that often are abnormally stretched (and therefore weak in their inner ranges). You can test clients' ability to hold the inner range of the deep abdominals (1) by assessing their abilities to hollow the abdomen, and (2) by monitoring lumbar lordosis and pelvic tilt while overloading the stability system. You can assess both actions by accurate palpation and motion recording, but I recommend use of pressure biofeedback, which will make the assessment considerably easier. Note that the pressure biofeedback unit is more useful for assessment rather than for continuing exercises.

To assess limb function relative to lumbar-pelvic stability, you can use a number of starting positions—two of which I will describe in detail.

Prone Abdominal Hollowing Test
Using Pressure Biofeedback

GOAL *To assess client's ability to hold the inner range of the deep abdominals.*

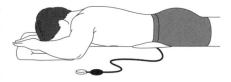

With your subject lying prone, place the pressure biofeedback unit beneath his abdomen with the upper edge of the device's bladder below his navel. Inflate the unit to 70 mm Hg, and instruct your client to perform abdominal hollowing (see chapter 4). The aim is to reduce the pressure reading on the biofeedback unit by 6-10 mm Hg

continued

Prone Abdominal Hollowing Test Using Pressure Biofeedback, continued

and to be able to maintain this contraction for 10 repetitions of 10 seconds each while breathing normally (Richardson and Hodges 1996).

Heel Slide Maneuver Using Pressure Biofeedback

GOAL *Assess the deep abdominals' ability to maintain spinal stability.*

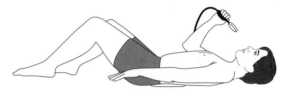

The subject begins in a crook lying position with the spine in a neutral position and the pressure biofeedback unit positioned beneath his lower spine. While you palpate the anterior superior iliac spine (ASIS), instruct him to gradually straighten one leg, sliding the heel along the ground to take the weight off the limb. During this action, the hip flexors are working eccentrically and pulling on the pelvis and lumbar spine. If the strong pull of these muscles is sufficient to displace the pelvis, you will be able to feel the pelvis tilt; moreover, the pressure shown on the dial of the biofeedback unit will change. If your client cannot complete the action without any alteration of pelvic tilt or depth of lordosis, palpate the abdominal muscle action. Often subjects will substitute their rectus abdominis and/or external oblique in an attempt to fix the pelvis rather than using transversus abdominis and internal oblique. Where this is the case, these deeper abdominal muscles will need to be re-educated.

Assessing Shortened Muscles

Mobilizer muscles have a tendency to tighten. Tightness in the hamstrings (mobilizers), for example, is common, while tightness in the gluteals (stabilizers) is rare. In addition to reducing range of motion, muscle tightening may lead to development of **trigger points** (Travell and Simmons 1983)—small hypersensitive regions within a muscle that stimulate afferent nerve fibers, causing pain. The sensation created is a deep tenderness with an overlying increase in tone, creating a palpably tender band of muscle. When palpated deeply, the trigger point creates a local muscle spasm, the "jump sign" (Janda 1993). Because tight muscles have a lowered irritability threshold, they are activated earlier than normal in a movement sequence—and they have less slack to take up before contraction begins. In addition, tight muscles have increased afferent input via the stretch receptors (Sahrmann 1990).

There are several important reasons why you should assess the tightness of your client's mobilizer muscles. First, since limited range of motion may not allow sufficient movement for correct body segment alignment, limbs may be pulled into positions that stress joint surfaces and collateral ligaments. Second, tightness in a muscle may, through reciprocal innervation, inhibit the opposing muscle through the process of pseudoparesis (Janda 1986). Third, stability must be relative to flexibility. Consider the straight-leg raise (SLR) exercise (see page 109): poor stability can lead the pelvis to tilt very early in the range of motion. Normally, the pelvis only tilts when the hamstring muscles reach the end of their stretch—they are fully 'wound up'—and this may not occur until 80-90° hip flexion. If pelvic tilt is seen before this (in a flexible individual), an imbalance exists. The individual's level of stability is not sufficient for her level of flexibility—she has lost active muscular control over a portion of her total range of motion, a fundamental feature in the difference between hypermobility and instability.

If you find muscle tightness, you can use the test movements as starting positions for stretching. But before prescribing stretching exercises, be sure that they will not place excessive strain on adjacent body parts because of relative stiffness. Your clients often will require some stability work before beginning the stretches. The need for stability work is indicated if the subject's alignment is degraded (partially lost) as a stretch is applied.

To assess tightness in those muscles that are most likely to exacerbate lower back problems, there are four principal tests—each of which in its own way will help you to assess restriction of pelvic motion: (1) the modified Thomas test, (2) the straight-leg raise (SLR) test, (3) the Ober test, and (4) the tripod test. Carefully note whether any of the movements in these tests reproduces the pain for which the patient has sought treatment; note also if the range is significantly less than the optimal position. (For the Thomas test, optimum is for the femur of the lower leg to drop down to the horizontal, and the tibia of the same leg to drop to the vertical. For the SLR, the optimal value is 70-80° from the horizontal; and for the Ober test, the upper leg should drop down to the level of the couch.) In either case, the muscle will require specific stretching.

The Thomas Test

GOAL *To assess/correct tightness in the iliopsoas and rectus femoris.*

The patient begins in crook lying at the end of the examination table. Instruct her to lift both knees up to her chest, keeping her back flattened

continued

The Thomas Test, continued

to a point where the sacrum just begins to lift away from the examination table surface, but not farther. You can monitor the movement of the pelvis and lumbar spine using a pressure biofeedback unit. As she holds one leg close to the chest to maintain the pelvic position, have her lower the other leg over the end of the table, maintaining a 90° angle at the knee (a). Optimal alignment occurs with the femur horizontal and aligned with the sagittal plane (no abduction) and with the subject's shoulder, hip, and knee more or less in line. The tibia should hang vertically (90° knee flexion) and be aligned with the sagittal plane (no hip rotation—see c). If the femur rests above the horizontal and the knee is flexed less than 90°, tightness may be present in either the iliopsoas or rectus femoris. If the rectus is tight, straightening the knee will take the stretch off the muscle and the leg will drop down (b). If the knee is straightened and the leg stays in place, it indicates tightness in the iliopsoas. Use palpation to distinguish between the psoas and iliacus. Psoas can be palpated deep in the abdomen at the side of the lumbar spine. Iliacus is found on the inner side of the pelvis. Both muscles take experience to palpate, as they lie beneath the abdominal contents (see figure 3.10b, page 58).

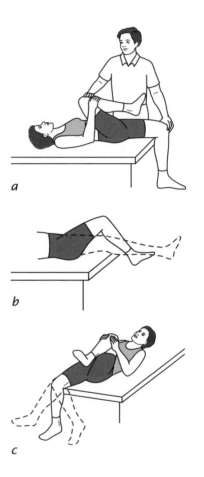

a

b

c

The Ober Test

GOAL *To assess both the length of tensor fasciae lata muscle and the tightness of the iliotibial band.*

The modified Ober test begins in side lying with the pelvis in a neutral position (a). Have your client bend her lower leg to improve overall body

continued

The Ober Test, continued

stability while you stabilize the pelvis to avoid lateral pelvic dipping. The examination table should be low enough to allow you to place pressure through the subject's iliac crest in the direction of the lower shoulder. You may monitor the position of the spine and pelvis using pressure biofeedback. While she maintains the neutral pelvic position, have your client abduct the upper leg to 15° above the horizontal and then extend her hip about 15°. She should then adduct it while maintaining extension. For an athlete, optimal muscle length would be confirmed if she is able to lower the upper leg to the level of the table; the nonathlete should be able to lower the leg to the horizontal (b). A false reading is obtained if the pelvis is allowed to tip and the lumbar spine to laterally flex. You can still proceed with the test when hip extension is limited, but you should further assess the hip tightness to determine if it results from muscular, capsular, or osteological factors—an examination for which you should refer the subject to an orthopedic physical therapist.

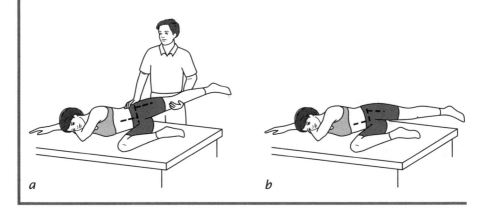

a   *b*

The Straight-Leg Raise (SLR) Test

GOAL *To assess tightness in hamstrings.*

Have your client lie supine on the examination table, one leg slightly bent. Have her raise the other leg while keeping it completely straight. Palpate the anterior rim of the pelvis to note the point at which the pelvis begins to posteriorly tilt due to hamstring tightness—this is the point at which a stable base is no longer being provided for the hamstrings to stretch against. Two body segments are moving here; this is a prime example of relative flexibility, as mentioned on page 95. As the maximal

continued

The Straight-Leg Raise (SLR) Test, continued

range of hamstring flexibility is reached, the pelvis will begin to tilt posteriorly, bringing the ischial tuberosity of the pelvis forward in an attempt to reduce tension in the hamstrings. Look for pelvic tilt, which will occur before the hamstrings are fully stretched to their end range. For example, if your client can stretch the hamstrings to 90° hip flexion, does the pelvis move at 80-90° as it should because the tension in the hamstrings is maximal? Or does the pelvis begin to tilt at perhaps 40-50°, when the tension in the hamstrings is only moderate? The latter case indicates a lack of muscular control over the pelvis—

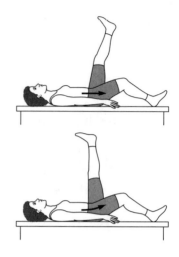

the individual is unable to create the stable pelvic base (using the trunk stabilizers) for the stretched hamstrings to pull against.

The Tripod Test

GOAL *To assess/correct imbalanced hamstrings.*

Have your client sit on the examination table with his lumbar spine in the neutral position and his feet hanging off the edge. As he straightens one leg, note two measures: (1) the point at which posterior pelvic tilting occurs, and (2) the total range of combined motion

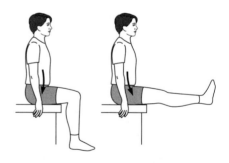

at both hip and knee. For optimal performance, the lumbar spine should remain neutral and should allow the knee to straighten to within 10° of full extension while the femur remains horizontal.

If you find muscle tightness, you can use the test movements as starting positions for stretching.

PRINCIPLES OF MUSCLE STRETCHING

Five methods of stretching are generally recognized: ballistic, static, active, and two PNF (proprioceptive neuromuscular facilitation) techniques (table 5.3). PNF stretching has been adopted by the sporting world from neurological physiotherapy treatments. By alternately contracting and relaxing muscles, these techniques capitalize on various muscle reflexes to achieve a greater level of relaxation during the stretch. The back stability program uses two PNF techniques: contract-relax (CR), and contract-relax-agonist-contract (CRAC). PNF stretching was believed at one time to be the most effective type of stretching (Etnyre and Abraham 1986; Holt and Smith 1983), with CRAC methods generally being better than CR. The data are not consistent, however. Moore and Kukulka (1991) found CRAC to cause more pain than either CR or static stretching; moreover, they found that static stretching appeared to be the most effective of all the techniques, leading to less pain and more range of motion. I recommend that you select stretching techniques on a client-by-client basis. Test to see what works best for each individual. The advantage of static stretching, of course, is that it does not require your presence or that of anyone else.

Table 5.3 Principal Stretching Techniques

Method	Action
▪ Ballistic	▪ Rapid jerking actions at end of range to force the tissues to stretch.
▪ Static	▪ Slowly and passively stretching the muscle to full range, and maintaining this stretched position for a set period—usually from 15 to 30 seconds.
▪ Active	▪ Contracting the agonist muscle to full inner range to impart a stretch on the antagonist.
▪ Contract-relax (CR)	▪ Isometrically contracting the stretched muscle, then relaxing and passively stretching the muscle still farther. This action is usually performed by a partner.
▪ Contract-relax-agonist-contract (CRAC)	▪ The same as CR, except that during the final stages of the stretching phase, the muscle opposite the one being stretched is contracted.

Here are the basic five stretching methods:

1. **Ballistic stretching** involves taking the limb to the end of its movement range and adding repetitive bouncing movements. This method is increasingly out of favor since it appears that it may cause injury and muscle soreness (Etnyre and Lee 1987). Although not recommended for regular training, ballistic stretching may have a place in the final stages of rehabilitation for athletes whose sport *requires* ballistic actions (e.g., high kicks in martial arts practice) (Norris 1998).

2. During **static stretching**, a muscle is stretched to the point of slight discomfort and held there for an extended period. A holding time of 30 seconds has been shown to be optimal, with 15 seconds being less effective and 60 seconds being not more effective (Bandy and Irion 1994). Repeating the stretch is important, with the greatest stretching effects occurring within the first four repetitions (Taylor et al. 1990). Easily remembered, basic guidelines for static stretching are 5 repetitions, holding each for 30 seconds, with a 30-second rest period between each movement.

3. **Active stretching** involves pulling a limb into full inner range so that the antagonist muscle is stretched passively while the agonist is strengthened. This type of stretch can be important when correcting muscle imbalance. The inner-range contraction helps shorten a lengthened (lax) muscle, while the shortened muscle is stretched using a functionally relevant movement. Webright et al. (1997) found static and active stretching equally effective when used daily for a six-week period. Static stretching involves less coordination and fewer repetitions than active stretching, so it is more appropriate to early treatment stages. Active stretching involves more complex coordination and requires greater segmental control, making it more useful in later stages of rehabilitation.

4. The **CR (contract-relax) PNF** technique involves lengthening a muscle until a comfortable stretch is felt. From this position, the muscle is isometrically contracted and held for a set period. The muscle is relaxed again, then taken to a new lengthened position until the subject again feels the full stretch. The rationale behind the CR method is that the contracted muscle will relax as a result of autogenic inhibition, as the Golgi tendon organ (GTO) fires to inhibit tension. Some authors argue that a maximal isometric contraction is needed to initiate relaxation through the GTO mechanism (Janda 1992). Others recommend the use of minimal isometric contractions (Lewit 1991), which seem more appropriate in situations where pain is present. A window of opportunity exists after isometric muscle contraction—since the stretch reflex is suppressed for about 10 seconds following isometric contraction (Moore and Kukulka 1991), the stretch must be imposed during this time.

5. With the **CRAC (contract-relax-agonist-contract) PNF** technique, the muscle is stretched as just described—but in the final stages of the stretch,

the opposing muscle groups are isometrically contracted to make use of reciprocal inhibition of the agonist and to reduce its tension.

To illustrate each of these procedures, consider stretching the hamstrings.

1. A *ballistic stretch* could involve keeping the leg straight while standing and vigorously reaching for the toes with a bouncing action. While the rapid action may actually tighten the muscle by increasing its tone, it may stretch other soft tissues—including the noncontractile muscle elements, muscle tendons, and ligaments surrounding the hip, knee, and spine. In this particular exercise, moreover, repeated spinal flexion may increase intradiscal pressure within the lumbar discs, potentially leading to discal migration (McKenzie 1981) or discal herniation. For this reason, ballistic stretching should only be performed in the presence of good lumbar stability and optimal segmental alignment.

2. An easy *static stretch* for the hamstrings involves lying supine on the floor in a doorway, with the hips just inside the door frame. With the leg farthest from the door frame flat on the ground and the back in neutral position, raise the other leg, keeping it straight, until it rests on the door frame. To increase/decrease the stretch, move the body closer to or farther away from the door frame. The stretch is held for 30 seconds.

3. An *active stretch* could be performed by standing, holding on to a wall bar for support, and lifting the straight leg upward using the force of the hip flexors.

4. An individual could perform the *CR technique* for the hamstrings while lying on his back. A training partner lifts his leg, keeping the knee straight. After holding the stretch for 10 seconds, the athlete contracts his hamstrings by pulling the straight leg down toward the floor against his partner's resistance. He holds the tension for 10 to 20 seconds—sufficient time to allow the GTO to override the stretch reflex. He then releases the tension, and the training partner reapplies the stretch.

5. The *CRAC technique* takes this stretch even further: as the stretch is applied, the athlete tries to increase the stretch himself by pulling the straight leg up toward his head, tensing his hip flexors. In so doing, the hamstrings are relaxed still further through reciprocal inhibition, and the stretch becomes even more effective.

STRETCHING TARGET MUSCLES

Several mobilizer muscles within the lumbar-pelvic region are commonly tight and may require stretching. It is generally best to begin with passive static stretching, followed by contract-relax techniques. Finally, the opposing muscles are shortened to full inner range to stretch the antagonist *actively*.

Thomas Test Stretch

GOAL *To stretch the hip flexors.*

This stretch is performed from the Thomas test position (see page 107). Any firm surface may be used at home, such as a sturdy coffee table. Your client should hold one knee tightly to her chest and allow the other leg to rest in a stretched position near the horizontal. To increase the emphasis on the rectus femorus muscle, the knee of the lower (horizontal) leg may be bent. Throughout the movement the back must remain flat on the table and the pelvis must not be allowed to move. She should hold the stretched position for 10-20 seconds, and then lower the leg slowly. Raising into the stretch position and recovering from it should be performed with control, taking 5 seconds in each direction. Reverse the legs and repeat the cycle two more times. Have her perform this stretch daily until she can perform the Thomas test satisfactorily.

Half Lunge

GOAL *To stretch the hip flexors.*

Have your client take up the half-kneeling position, with one hand on a chair to aid balance and the other hand pressing into the lumbar spine on the side of the dependent leg (the one with the knee on the floor). Instruct him to keep his abdomen hollowed throughout the exercise in order to keep the lumbar spine in neutral position. Tell him to lunge his body forward, forcing the dependent hip into extension while avoiding increasing the lordosis. Hold this stretched position for 10 seconds.

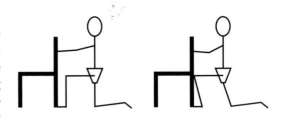

Instruct your client to perform this exercise three times a day, each session comprising 10 lunges on each side.

Hip Hitch

GOAL *To work the trunk side flexors on the side of the weight-bearing leg. This exercise is used in preparation for the Ober stretch, to enable the subject to control the pelvis with the trunk side flexors.*

Your client should stand with her hands on a tabletop for support at home, or a bar in the clinic. Instructing her to keep her legs straight throughout the movement, have her make one leg shorter than the other by laterally tilting her pelvis. It may help by suggesting that she imagine she is drawing the rim of her pelvis vertically upward on the side of the shortening leg, raising her heel slightly off the ground. To avoid simply coming up onto the toes, have your client dorsiflex (pull up) her foot—this way you 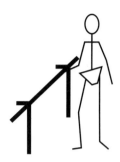 can assess movement of the whole leg in one section. Tell her to keep her upper body from swaying and to relax her shoulders. Once she has mastered this action, have her practice it unsupported (hand off the tabletop), then lying supine, and finally while lying on her side. In each case, the knee must be kept straight throughout the movement, with the action coming from pelvic movement alone.

When using the side lying position, she should place her upper hand on her upper hip to provide resistance (since there is no gravity to resist), and she should pull her upper leg up as she simultaneously pushes the leg that is against the floor down (as if she's trying to make that leg as long as possible).

Instruct your client to perform this exercise three times a day, with five repetitions for each side from each of the three starting positions (standing, supine, side lying).

Ober Test Stretch

GOAL *Stretch the iliotibial band (ITB) and tensor fasciae lata (TFL).*

The ITB and TFL can become overactive and tight to compensate for a weak or inactive gluteus medius muscle. When this occurs, tightness in the ITB-TFL can cause friction of this structure over the greater trochanter of the femur or the lateral epicondyle of the femur. Both of these areas

continued

Ober Test Stretch, continued

are common sites for *ITB friction syndrome* a common overuse condition, particularly among distance runners, that results from muscle imbalance.

Beginning in a side-lying position, your client first performs the hip hitch as just described. Then he continues with the Ober test actions (see page 108): he abducts the upper leg to 15° above the horizontal, extends it to 15°, then lowers it into adduction (toward the floor or couch) *while maintaining an immobile pelvis*. The exercise is complex because it requires the control of two body parts simultaneously. Supervise your client closely, (1) watching the pelvic rim to note any unwanted pelvic movement and (2) noting if the hip extension is being maintained. When the hip extension is lost, the leg falls forward into flexion and the stretch is lost from the TFL. If your client is unable to maintain stability of his pelvis, assist him by holding the pelvis in place with your hands.

Active Knee Extension, Holding Thigh

GOAL *To stretch the hamstrings.*

Have your client lie supine, then raise one leg to 90° hip flexion, comfortably bent at the knee, and hold it with her hands beneath the thigh. Then instruct her to straighten the leg as much as possible. The sensation should be one of a deep stretching sensation rather than acute pain. The 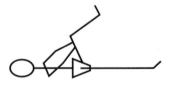 discomfort should reduce as the stretch is held. She should hold the stretch for 30 seconds. Instruct her to perform this stretch at home three times a day, with two repetitions for each leg at each session.

Active Knee Extension, Pushing Against Thigh

GOAL *To strengthen hip flexors, hip extensors, and hamstrings.*

This action stretches the hamstrings while activating the quadriceps against a resistance. Increasing the quadriceps activity should reduce the hamstring tone through reciprocal innervation.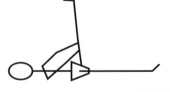

continued

Active Knee Extension, Pushing Against Thigh, continued

Have your client lie supine and, with one knee comfortably bent, raise that leg until it is at a 60° angle to the floor. Instruct him then to straighten the leg, and then slowly raise the straightened leg till it is vertical (90° hip flexion). He should keep the leg completely straight and use only his hip flexor muscles to raise the leg (no use of the hands this time!), without allowing the knee to bend. Once the leg is vertical (or as near vertical as your client can raise it), have him place his hand on the leg just above the knee and use it as a fulcrum to straighten the leg just a little bit more. This is especially helpful in stretching the hamstrings. He should hold this position for 30 seconds.

Tell your client to do this exercise three times a day, using three repetitions for each leg per session.

Tripod Stretch

GOAL *To stretch the hamstrings.*

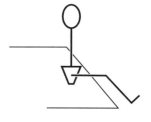

Have your client sit upright on the edge of a table, her lumbar spine in its neutral position, her feet hanging over the edge of the table. She should maintain abdominal hollowing throughout the exercise. Have her straighten one leg, to stretch the hamstrings against the stable base of the unmoving pelvis. She should hold the leg straight for 15 seconds, then slowly lower it.

Instruct your client to perform this exercise three times a day, with three repetitions per leg per session.

Trunk Side Flexor Stretch

GOAL *To stretch the quadratus lumborum and lateral portion of the oblique abdominals.*

These muscles are commonly tight after prolonged periods of sitting or bed rest. Have your client stand with his back against a wall, his feet shoulder-width apart, his hands clasped behind the head. He should keep his abdomen hollowed throughout the exercise. Instruct him to slowly bend his spine (and *only* his spine) to one side, being very careful to *keep his pelvis level* and his knees straight. Until he learns what the

continued

Trunk Side Flexor Stretch, continued

proper movement feels like, you should place your hands on his pelvis and let him know when it's bending. Tell him to reach his upper elbow as far toward the ceiling as he can, in an attempt to "lengthen his spine," and to hold this position for 30 seconds. Then he should repeat the exercise to the other side. The height of the upper elbow indicates the range of motion obtained, and the comparative range of each side will reveal your client's degree of symmetry.

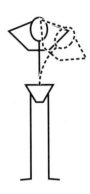

Instruct your client to do this stretch three times a day on each side.

Four-Point Kneeling Stretch

GOAL *To stretch the erector spinae.*

The erector spinae muscles also can tighten during long periods of sitting or bed rest. Have your client assume a 4-point kneeling position. Emphasize that, throughout this exercise, she must move only her spine, with

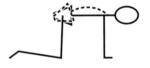

her shoulders remaining over her hands and her hips remaining over her knees at all times. Have her tilt her pelvis posteriorly and continue flexing her spine until her face points toward the groin. She should hold this position for 30 seconds, then slowly relax back toward the starting position.

Instruct your client to perform this exercise three times a day, with six repetitions per session.

SUMMARY

- Muscles can be divided roughly, although not unambiguously, into stabilizer or mobilizer muscles.
- Stabilizer muscles tend to be deep, to contain mainly slow-twitch fibers, to control only one joint, and primarily to *prevent* movement while stabilizing a joint. They are the primary postural muscles.
- Mobilizer muscles tend to be more superficial, to contain mainly fast-twitch fibers, to act over two joints, and primarily to *create* movement.

- Disuse, long-term bed rest, and injury can cause muscle systems to become imbalanced—with an agonist shortened while its antagonist is stretched.

- To train specific muscles, you must carefully target those muscles in your exercise prescriptions; exercises meant to improve back stability often fail to do so because they target the wrong muscles (especially the deep stabilizer muscles).

- You can treat such imbalance by prescribing exercises that strengthen/ shorten the stretched muscle and stretch the shortened muscle; this chapter describes a number of such exercises.

6

Basic Abdominal Muscle Training

Much of the back stability program involves working on the abdominal muscles. Especially for your clients who want to take abdominal training further (to enhance performance rather than merely to build stability), you must offer training that is both safe and effective. First I want to discuss currently popular abdominal exercises and assess their effects on the muscles and tissue. Then I will present modifications to improve the safety and effectiveness of such exercises.

CURRENT PRACTICE IN ABDOMINAL TRAINING

Abdominal training can be dangerous, whether for competitive sport or for general fitness. In sport, athletes often adhere with almost religious fervor to traditional but potentially harmful training methods. In the general population, fashion often dictates which movements are in favor— yet many popular exercises lack reliable scientific foundation. Before you can prescribe the most appropriate trunk exercises for your clients, you must understand what the traditional exercises actually achieve. To this end I will begin by briefly analyzing the two major categories of abdominal exercises: the *sit-up* and the *leg raise.*

The Sit-Up

In the **sit-up,** an individual comes from a supine lying to a long sitting position using hip flexion, usually combined with trunk flexion.

In a classic sit-up, the rectus abdominis shows activity as soon as the head lifts (Walters and Partridge 1957), and as a consequence the rib cage is depressed anteriorly. This initial period of flexion emphasizes the supraumbilical portion of the rectus; the infraumbilical portion contracts later, with the internal oblique (Kendall et al. 1993). As the internal oblique contracts, it pulls on the lower ribs, increasing the infrasternal angle by causing the ribs to flare out.

Fixation of the pelvis is provided by the hip flexors, especially the iliacus through its attachment to the pelvic rim. The strong pull of the hip flexors is partially counteracted by the pull of the lateral fibers of external oblique and the infraumbilical portion of the rectus abdominis, which tend to tilt the pelvis posteriorly. Action of the external oblique, if powerful enough, compresses the ribs and reduces the infrasternal angle once more (Kendall et al. 1993).

Problems Resulting From Poor Conditioning

Initiation of the sit-up action sometimes leads to "bow stringing" in poorly toned individuals. For the superficial abdominals (rectus abdominis and external oblique) to pull flat, the deep abdominals (transversus abdominis and internal oblique) must be able to pull on the rectus sheath to hold the abdominal wall down. Many people, however, have lost the ability to coordinate action of both the superficial and deep abdominals, which this action requires—the two sets of abdominal muscles are imbalanced, with poorly recruited deep abdominals and dominant superficial abdominals. When this is the case, the abdominal wall appears to *dome* and the athlete may lift the trunk with the lumbar spine extended or flat rather than flexed (figure 6.1).

> **KEY POINT:** Weak deep abdominal muscles cannot hold the rectus abdominis down as it contracts, leading to "doming" of the abdominal wall.

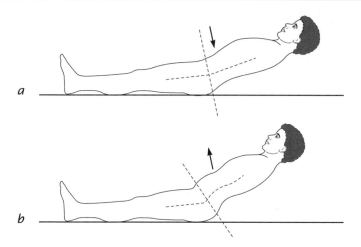

Figure 6.1 Trunk alignment during a sit-up exercise. *(a)* Strong deep abdominals flatten abdominal wall. *(b)* Weakened deep abdominals allow abdominal wall "doming," while lengthened superficial abdominals allow anterior pelvic tilt and hollowing of the back.
From Norris 1998.

Poorly conditioned subjects also tend to use the hip extensors to momentarily tilt the pelvis posteriorly at the beginning of a sit-up, prestretching the hip flexors. This gives the hip flexors a mechanical advantage before hip flexion occurs and reduces both the work required of the abdominals and the conditioning effect of the exercise on the abdominals.

During this phase, the abdominal muscles work eccentrically (Ricci et al. 1981).

Effects of Foot Fixation

If a person attempts a sit-up from the supine position without allowing trunk flexion, the legs tend to lift up from the supporting surface—this occurs because the legs constitute roughly one-third of total body weight whereas the trunk contributes two-thirds.

The upper body's center of gravity moves toward the hip as the abdominal muscles flex the spine, reducing the lever arm of the trunk and enabling the subject to perform the sit-up without lifting the legs (figure 6.2).

When the abdominal muscles are weak and lengthened, maximum spinal flexion does not occur because the muscles are unable to pull the lumbar spine into full inner range—the lever arm of the trunk remains long, and the legs lift. The point at which this occurs in the movement depends on a subject's weight and height.

If the feet are fixed, however, the hip flexors can pull powerfully without causing the legs to lift. The act of foot fixation itself, in fact, may facilitate the iliopsoas (Janda and Schmid 1980). To pull against the fixation point, one must use active dorsiflexion—which simulates the gait pattern at heel contact, increasing activity in the tibialis anterior, quadriceps, and iliopsoas (a pattern known as **flexor synergy during gait**) (Atkinson 1986).

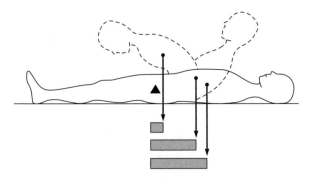

Figure 6.2 As the trunk flexes, the center of gravity of the upper body moves caudally.
From Norris 1998.

KEY POINT: The hip flexor muscles contract powerfully in a traditional sit-up. Fixing the foot causes the hip flexors to work even harder, without significantly increasing the work on the abdominal muscles.

The Straight-Leg Raise

The bilateral straight-leg raise (SLR) creates only slight activity in the upper rectus, although the lower rectus contributes a greater proportion of the total abdominal work in this exercise than with the sit-up (Lipetz and Gutin 1970). The rectus works isometrically to fix the pelvis against the strong pull of iliopsoas (Silvermetz 1990). The iliopsoas contracts with maximum force when the lever arm of the leg is greatest (near the horizontal) and reduces as the leg is lifted toward the vertical.

Problems Resulting From Poor Conditioning

In subjects with weaker abdominals, the pelvis tilts and the lumbar spine hyperextends during the SLR. This forced hyperextension dramatically increases stress on the facet joints, especially those in the lumbar spine. The movement is likely to be limited by impaction of the inferior articular processes on the laminae of the vertebrae below (see chapter 2) or, in some cases, by contact between the spinous processes (Twomey and Taylor 1987). Rapid action of this kind can damage the facet joint structures. Once the facet and lamina are touching each other, further loading causes axial rotation of the superior vertebra (Yang and King 1984); the superior vertebra then pivots, causing the inferior articular process to move backward, overstretching the joint capsule.

Effects of Arm Fixation

When the legs are lifted in an SLR, the body position is less secure because its base of support is smaller. People tend to rock toward the side of the lifted leg (where one leg is lifted) or to struggle to keep their backs on the floor (where both legs are lifted). Fixing the arms by holding onto an overhead object (e.g., gym bench) with the arms, or by pressing down with the flats of the hands with the arms by the side, improves the security of the starting position.

The disadvantage of fixing the arms, however, is that people can pull harder with their hip flexors without realizing they have lost their lumbar alignment. This is especially true of the bilateral leg raise action. At the beginning of this action the leverage from the legs is maximal, as they are horizontal. Without fixing their arms, poorly conditioned subjects may be unable to lift their legs at all—thereby self-limiting potential stress on the lumbar spine. With arms fixed, however, they may be able to lift their legs by rapidly pulling with their arms and "jerking" their legs up with a rapid contraction of the hip flexors. Once the legs move toward the vertical, their leverage is reduced and the movement can be continued—leading people to believe (wrongly) that, since they completed the action, they must have performed it correctly. The jerking action is extremely dangerous, however, due to the compression and shear forces it imposes on the lumbar spine.

For SLRs, then, permit your clients to fix their arms *only* when they will perform the exercises in a slow and controlled fashion, and *only* after you have chosen the exercise most appropriate for their specific body condition. Straight-leg actions are inappropriate for poorly conditioned subjects or for those with a history of back pain.

MODIFICATIONS OF TRADITIONAL ABDOMINAL EXERCISES

Your clients will find it easier to learn modifications of exercises they already know than to learn totally new procedures. Such modifications also may be more acceptable to "experienced trainers" than if you try to convince them to change their ways completely. Remember that in every case your clients should begin with their abdomens hollowed and their lumbar spines in neutral position. Except where otherwise noted, have your clients perform 8-10 reps of each exercise once a day, three days per week. Except where otherwise noted, the initial movement of each exercise should take about 2-3 seconds; your clients should hold the position for 1-3 seconds; then should perform the reverse movement in 2-3 seconds. Note, however, that these are mere guidelines. If at any time your clients are not working hard enough, increase the overload by slowing down the exercise or increasing the number of repetitions. If they are working too hard, reduce the overload.

As your clients become more proficient at a given exercise, they can increase the number of repetitions, perform the movements more slowly, and/ or increase the time for the holding period. Remember to emphasize to your clients that, when moving slowly, they must breathe normally (no holding their breaths!). The limiting factor is not how many times individuals can superficially perform an exercise—but rather how well they can do it *while still maintaining proper spinal alignment and abdominal hollowing.*

Modifications of the Sit-Up

Bending the knees and hips to alter the starting position of the sit-up affects both passive and active actions of the hip flexors, and the biomechanics of the lumbar spine. Supine lying stretches the iliopsoas, aligning it with the horizontal (figure 6.3). As the muscle contracts in this position, trunk lifting is at a mechanical disadvantage and vertebral compression is at its greatest—the ratio of lifting to compression is approximately 1:10 (Watson 1983). Flexing the knees pulls the iliopsoas more vertically, reducing the ratio of trunk lifting to vertebral compression to 2:5 in crook lying and 1:1 in bench lying.

If flexion historically has exacerbated clients' back pain (consult with their physical therapists on this), they can use fewer repetitions (2 or 3) while increasing the exercise timing (8-12 seconds in each direction). This schedule reduces the number of flexion movements but maintains the overload on the muscle.

With 45° hip flexion, tension in the iliopsoas is 70-80% of its maximum; with the hips and knees flexed to 90°, the figure reduces to 40-50% (Johnson and Reid 1991). Note, however, that the iliopsoas develop passive tension due to elastic recoil. Since the iliopsoas are not fully stretched when the hips are flexed, they cannot passively limit the posterior tilt of the pelvis. Instead, to fix the pelvis and provide a stable base for the abdominals to pull on when the hips are flexed, the hip flexors contract earlier in the sit-up action. This contraction has reduced intensity (Walters and Partridge 1957), however, due to the length-tension relationship of the muscle.

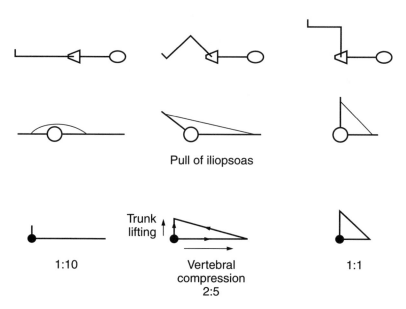

Figure 6.3 Flexing the hip lengthens the moment arm of the iliopsoas, enabling the muscle to complete the sit-up action with less force. Thus, vertebral compression is reduced.
From Norris 1998.

With the legs straight in the traditional sit-up position, the iliopsoas are stretched and can passively limit posterior tilting of the pelvis. The stretched position also enables the iliopsoas to exert greater force during hip flexion—which means that, if the abdominal muscles are too weak to maintain the position of the pelvis, the stronger hip flexors will hyperextend the lumbar spine and cause the pelvis to tilt forward, thus lengthening the abdominals and hyperextending the lumbar spine. This type of action is therefore unsuitable for postural re-education if the aim is to shorten lengthened abdominal muscles.

Bent Knee Sit-Up

GOAL *To strengthen the abdominals while reducing the action of the hip flexors.*

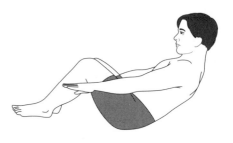

Have your client begin with the crook lying position, knees flexed to 90° and hips flexed to 45°. He should lift his trunk, moving from the hip alone, and either at the same time or slightly later should flex his hips. Suggest that he imagine himself as a hinge pivoting on the hip joint. The action must be slow and controlled, without strain. A pure bent knee sit-up requires keeping the spine straight, moving it around the fixed hip, and reducing the action of the hip flexors. Tell your client that, if he feels his back muscles straining instead of his abdominals, he should stop the exercise and perform abdominal hollowing before resuming the exercise.

Trunk Curl

GOAL *To shorten and strengthen the rectus abdominis.*

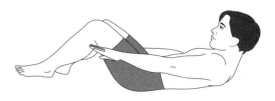

In this exercise there is no hip flexion, the lumbar spine remaining in contact with the supporting surface. Have your client assume the crook lying position, knees flexed to 90° and hips flexed to 45°.

continued

Trunk Curl, continued

Instruct him to "roll through the spine," performing cervical flexion until the chin comes toward the chest, followed by thoracic flexion, until only the lumbar spine remains on the supporting surface. He then should reverse these actions, first lowering the thoracic spine from bottom to top and finally releasing the cervical spine so that the head is gently lowered back onto the supporting surface.

Bench Curl

GOAL *To strengthen the upper abdominals (supraumbilical portion of rectus abdominis with the lateral fibers of external oblique) while reducing the pull of the hip flexors and lessening the stresses on the lumbar spine.*

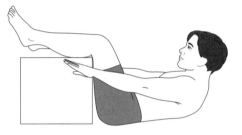

The bench curl is performed from a starting position of 90° flexion at both the hip and the knee, with the calves supported on a bench or chair. Since shortening the hip flexors in this way reduces their ability to contribute to the movement, hip flexor action does not obscure the action of the abdominals. Instruct your client to "roll through the spine" just as in the trunk curl.

Modifications of the Straight-Leg Raise

As none of the abdominal muscles actually crosses the hip, these muscles are not prime movers for the SLR. The SLR is nevertheless important for abdominal training because it enhances the pelvic stabilizing function of the infraumbilical portion of the rectus abdominis and lateral external oblique.

Several modifications of the bilateral straight-leg raise can help reduce stress on the lumbar spine.

Heel Slide (see also discussion of this action in chapter 8)

GOAL *To statically overload the abdominal muscles, increasing the emphasis on the deep abdominals.*

Have your client assume a crook lying position, then straighten one leg while keeping the heel on the ground and sliding the leg into extension. Instruct her to place her hands over her lower abdomen on either side of the navel, her fingertips 5-6 inches apart. She should perform abdominal hollowing and keep the abdominal muscles tight beneath her hands as she slowly performs the leg action over a period of about 3-5 seconds (see page 170).

Leg Lowering

GOAL *To increase the static overload on the abdominal muscles while maintaining a neutral spine.*

Instruct your client to lie supine with hips flexed to 90° but with the knees extended so that the straightened legs are vertical. Tell him to slowly lower his legs until the pelvis begins to tilt. As soon as this occurs, he should raise the legs again to 90° hip flexion. Each cycle should take about 3-5 seconds. The advantage of this exercise over the standard straight-leg 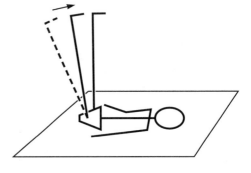 raise is one of changing leverage. With the standard leg raising action, the subject starts with maximum leverage on the leg, forcing the hip flexors and abdominals to work maximally from the very beginning. With leg lowering, the starting position provides minimum leverage. As the legs are lowered away from the vertical, leverage increases—but the subject is able to *control* the descent of the legs and avoid the position of maximal leverage that would cause the spine to hyperextend. Should a client find the leg lowering difficult to control, tell him to bend his knees in order to reduce leverage on the leg; or have him perform the exercise close to a wall, so he cannot fully lower the legs.

Bench Lying Pelvic Raise

GOAL *To strengthen the abdominal muscles, especially the lower (infraumbilical) portion of rectus abdominis.*

Instruct your client to lie supine and flex both hips and knees 90°—a position she will maintain throughout the movement. She should place her arms by her sides, hands flat on the table or floor. Have her lift her buttocks from the ground by flexing her lumbar spine, while keeping her legs relatively inactive. Although in this movement the lumbar spine is flexed as with 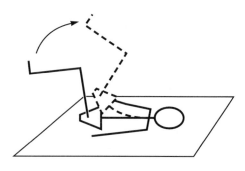 the trunk curl, the movement occurs from "below upward" with the L5-S1 joint moving first followed by flexion of each successively higher lumbar segment. The trunk curl provides the reverse movement (above downward) (McKenzie 1981).

Wall Bar Hanging Leg Raise

GOAL *To strengthen the lower rectus, with increasing leg leverage, while providing traction for the lumbar spine.*

Performing leg raises while hanging from a wall bar considerably reduces the leverage forces on the lumbar spine and provides traction. Explain to your client that he must hold a neutral pelvic position throughout all versions of this exercise, preventing anterior tilt of the pelvis, and (except in the last variation) pressing the small of his back into the wall bars. There are three forms of the exercise:

1. Instruct your client to stand with his back against the wall bar, place his arms overhead, and hold onto a bar above head height. Then, avoiding any jerking action, he should slowly take his weight onto his arms and, keeping his legs straight, raise his feet slightly off the ground (a). Tell him to feel the stretch through the whole of his spine—and to tighten his abdominal muscles while pressing his lower back into the wall bar and breathing normally. Instruct him to hold this position for 2-3 seconds, and then release it slowly.

continued

Wall Bar Hanging Leg Raise, continued

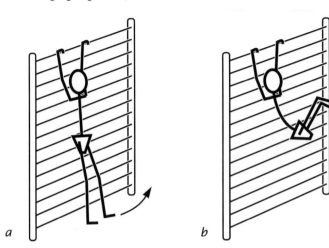

2. The action then progresses to include hip and knee flexion. For this exercise, instruct your client to bend his knees and raise them until he has achieved 90° hip flexion (i.e., knees level with hips), while still keeping the lumbar spine in contact with the wall bars. Be sure that he doesn't jerk his knees up—the movement should be slow, lasting about 3-5 seconds. Suggest that he focus his attention on his abdominal muscles, pulling them in as he moves his legs. After holding the 90° flexed position for 2-3 seconds, he should slowly lower his legs to the starting position.

3. The final progression of this exercise requires flexing the lumbar spine to lift the back away from the support of the wall bars. This action, while working the abdominals hard, also strengthens and possibly shortens the hip flexors. Once your client has reached the 90° flexed position as in the previous exercise, instruct him to round his spine in order to slowly lift his tailbone away from the wall bar (b). Emphasize that, in the reverse movement, your client must not allow his body to "fall" and strike his tailbone hard onto the wall bar.

AB ROLLER EXERCISES

The ab roller can help your clients re-educate their muscles for the trunk curl action (spinal flexion) as distinct from the sit-up movement (straight spine moving on a fixed femur). The frame allows only trunk flexion, while the subject's lumbar spine remains in contact with the ground.

Basic Crunch

GOAL *To work the abdominal muscles in general, with increased emphasis on inner-range activity of the upper abdominals.*

Instruct your client to lie on her back with her knees bent and feet flat on the floor (crook lying), her head and neck on the neck rest of the machine. She should either grasp the centers of the curled handles at the sides of the device's arms or hold her arms straight with her wrists against the horizontal piece that connects the handles—whichever is more comfortable for her. Tell her to curl her trunk ("basic crunch"), keeping her 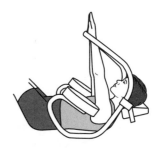 head on the pad and gently assisting the movement by extending the shoulder. Her focus should be on pulling the abdominal wall in (hollowing). There is a tendency with this exercise for people to rapidly "pump" the movement—an error that adds considerable momentum to the spine and may forcibly overstretch the posterior tissues. Make sure that the exercise stays slow and controlled, following the earlier-stated principle that each movement should last 2-3 seconds. With time, your client will gain sufficient control to rest her elbows on the machine pads and press down with her elbows (shoulder extension), gripping only lightly with her open hand on the machine frame.

Reverse Crunch

GOAL *Intense strengthening for the lower rectus abdominis.*

This action emphasizes the lower portion of rectus abdominis. Instruct your client to raise her legs (one at a time) into a vertical position and maintain this position throughout the exercise. The exercise action is to vertically lift the leg as though trying to reach the toes to the ceiling, while keeping the upper body still. In so doing, she will lift her sacrum from the floor, a movement which combines posterior pelvic tilt with lower lumbar flexion. The movement must be slow and controlled with no lunging or bouncing.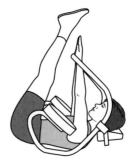

Double Crunch

GOAL *To strengthen the upper and lower rectus abdominis.*

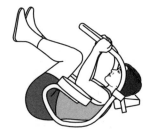

The double crunch movement combines the actions of the trunk curl and the leg raise, working both the upper and lower portions of the rectus abdominis. Since two body areas work together for this exercise, it requires a greater degree of coordination than the other crunches. Starting position is the same as that of the basic crunch. Instruct your client to simultaneously (1) raise her knees toward her chest, posteriorly tilting the pelvis; and (2) raise her upper body (as in the basic crunch) to flex the spine. The lumbar spine remains on the floor, while the shoulders and sacrum both lift off the floor. She should perform the action slowly and precisely, avoiding the excess momentum on the spine that rapid "pumping" actions cause. Make sure that she neither holds her breath nor hyperventilates (breathes too rapidly). If she does hyperventilate, she should rest on her side and not attempt to stand up until the lightheadedness has passed.

Side Crunch

GOAL *To strengthen the oblique abdominals while also working the rectus abdominis.*

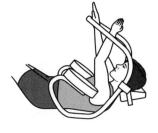

Have your client begin in the basic crunch position, then lower her knees to one side; she should raise her arms up straight and cross them, her wrists resting on the horizontal bar as in one version of the basic crunch. Instruct her to perform, from this altered starting position, the same actions as in the basic crunch—to curl her trunk, keeping her head on the pad. Since asymmetry is common in this body region, your client may find that one side is stronger or more flexible than the other; as she continues with this exercise (assuming she uses correct form), the asymmetry should resolve and both sides should perform equally.

SUMMARY

- Popular abdominal exercises can be only moderately effective, or even dangerous, for some people with lower back injuries.
- Poorly conditioned individuals tend to place emphasis on the wrong muscles to perform straight-leg raises and sit-ups; modified versions of these exercises force them to use the correct muscles.
- Poorly conditioned subjects, or those with a history of back pain, should avoid straight-leg abdominal exercises altogether.
- It is generally more productive for you to introduce your clients to modifications of exercises they already know than to try to teach them totally new movements.
- This chapter introduces specific abdominal exercises that are both safe and maximally effective for functional abdominal training.

7

Posture

Because postural alignment reflects changes in muscle length, it is the first form of assessment you will generally use to determine muscle imbalance. Before you can diagnose changes in alignment, however, you need a standard of optimal posture. The body moves continually around the optimal position in a process called *body sway*, and back stability is an essential component of this mechanism. In this chapter, I describe four principal types of posture.

OPTIMAL POSTURAL ALIGNMENT

Posture is the arrangement of body parts in a state of balance that protects the supporting structures of the body against injury or progressive deformity—a definition given in 1947 by the Posture Committee of the American Academy of Orthopaedic Surgeons (Cailliet 1983). A good posture is therefore effortless, nonfatiguing, and painless when the individual remains erect for reasonable periods (Cailliet 1981). Muscles function most efficiently in such an alignment, and the joints are optimally positioned (Bullock-Saxton 1988).

Optimal posture combines both minimal muscle work and minimal joint loading. It is the *combination* of these two factors that is important—where optimal posture is lost (for example in "slouched standing"), the muscle activity is clearly reduced, but there is a significant increase in joint loading.

Minimizing joint loading *over time* is important—articular cartilage gains its nutrition through intermittent loading (Norris 1998), and an even distribution of force is preferable to point pressure. Contact pressure is directly proportional to the transmitted force, but inversely proportional to area (McConnell 1993). Distributing force over a larger area by optimizing segmental alignment, therefore, reduces joint surface compression and lessens the risk of degenerative changes to a joint. The aim of any posture should be to reduce total energy expenditure and lessen stress on the supporting body structures.

KEY POINT: A good posture reduces total energy expenditure and lessens the stress on the supporting body structures.

Any change in the alignment of one body segment automatically causes neighboring segments to move in an attempt to maintain stability. If one body segment moves forward, for example, another must move backward to keep the line of gravity of the body (LOG) within the base of support (figure 7.1). Over time, changes in force per unit area cause tissue adaptation (Norkin and Levangie 1992). Changes in serial sarcomere number within muscles (see chapter 5), for example, are adaptations to postural changes over time. Shortening ligaments lead to reduced range of motion, while lengthening ligaments reduce a joint's passive stability.

Static posture—when the body is stationary—reflects the alignment of body segments and can reflect both changes in load distribution across joints and resting muscle length. Such postures include standing, sitting, and lying. **Dynamic posture**—body position during movement—can give information about body segment alignment, muscle actions, and motor skill. Typical dynamic postures are walking, running, jumping, and lifting. You can use both description of position (kinematic) and of force (kinetic) to assess posture.

POSTURAL STABILITY AND BODY SWAY

When standing erect, the human body has a small base of support due to its bipedal stance and comparatively high center of gravity (approximately

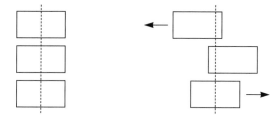

Figure 7.1 When one body segment moves out of alignment, a neighboring segment moves in the opposite direction to maintain the line of gravity within the base of support.

at the second sacral segment). Humans are thus relatively unstable in comparison with quadrupeds with their larger base of support and lower center of gravity. Maintaining an erect posture takes surprisingly little energy, however, as a result of constant motion brought about by postural control. This motion (postural sway) depends on kinesthesis, or "motion sense" (Kent 1994), which enables us to detect the position of our body parts through organs of proprioception, vision, the vestibular apparatus in the inner ear, and skin receptors. Normal postural sway consists of a small continuous motion in the sagittal plane. This oscillation of the center of gravity results from alternating muscle activity—possibly a relief mechanism to reduce lower-limb fatigue and to aid blood flow (Bullock-Saxton et al. 1991).

Excessive postural sway generally reveals poor balance and stability, a situation commonly seen in the elderly and inactive. Heavier people also may exhibit greater body sway (Sugano and Takeya 1970), as may taller individuals (Murray et al. 1975). Training usually can reduce postural sway. In the elderly, strength training may improve stability and limit postural sway (Hughes et al. 1996); following ankle injury, postural sway increases. By using balance and coordination training, body sway may be reduced to normal values once more (Bernier and Perrin 1998). Levels of postural sway can predict risk of recurrent falls among frail nursing home residents (Thapa et al. 1996). Lord and colleagues (1996) reduced fracture risk in women (ages 60-85) using a general aerobic exercise program whose effect was to improve postural sway rather than to change bone density.

BASIC POSTURAL ASSESSMENT

You can assess static posture through comparisons to a standard reference line (Kendall et al. 1993), which represents the line of gravity. A weight board can help identify both the center of gravity (COG) and the vertical extension of this point to the ground (line of gravity). Find the horizontal distance from the edge of the board to the subject's line of gravity (d) by multiplying the combined weight of subject and board by the total length of the board (L) and dividing the result by the subject's body weight (W). See Luttgens and Wells (1982) for full details of this method.

As the vertical extension of the COG, the LOG must pass within the body's base of support to maintain stability. The closer the body segments are to the LOG, the less torque there is around a joint. Where the LOG passes through the joint axis, no torque is created around that joint. If the LOG passes some distance from the joint axis, gravitational torque would tend to move the body segment *toward* the line of gravity were the segment not counterbalanced by elastic recoil of soft tissue and muscle action (Norkin and Levangie 1992). With the LOG anterior to the joint axis, the proximal segment of the body connected to the joint tends to move anteriorly (figure 7.2); posterior motion tends to occur when the LOG is posterior to the joint axis.

In the standard posture (viewed from the side), the subject is positioned with a **plumb line** representing the LOG, passing just in front of lateral malleolus (the bulge on the outside of the ankle). In an ideal posture, this line should pass just anterior to the midline of the knee and then through the greater trochanter, bodies of the lumbar vertebrae, shoulder joint, bodies of the cervical vertebrae, and the lobe of the ear (figure 7.3). Since the LOG is anterior to the ankle joint, gravity is continuously pulling the tibia anteriorly. This would result in enough dorsiflexion to unbalance the body were it not for constant opposing resistance provided by muscle action from the soleus (Norkin and Levangie 1992). The LOG passes in front of the knee joint axis (but behind the patella), forcing the femur anteriorly and creating an extension torque resisted by the posterior knee structures. Table 7.1 shows the gravitational torques created by the position of the LOG and the opposing structures resisting these torques.

When viewed from the front, with the feet 3-4 inches (10 cm) apart, the LOG should bisect the body into two equal halves. The anterior superior iliac spines (ASIS) should be approximately in the same horizontal plane, and the pubis and ASIS should be in the same vertical plane (Kendall et al. 1993). This alignment defines the neutral lumbar-pelvic alignment, which typically is about 5° to the horizontal. The joint axes of the hips, knees, and ankles should be equidistant from the LOG, and the LOG should transect the vertebral bodies (Norkin and Levangie 1992). The gravitational torque imposed on one side of the body should equal that of the other side.

Anatomical landmarks that provide comparisons for horizontal level on the right and left sides of the body include the knee creases, buttock

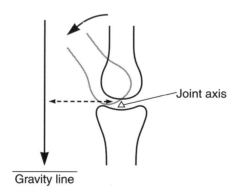

Figure 7.2 When the gravity line falls outside a joint, the proximal body segment tends to move toward the gravity line.

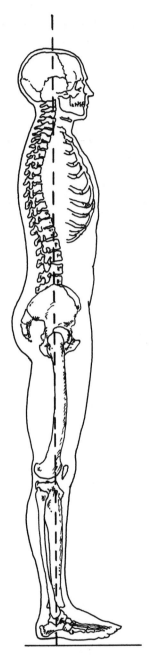

Figure 7.3 The standard reference line for posture.

creases, pelvic rim, inferior angle of the scapulae, acromion processes, ears, and the external occipital protuberances. You also can observe alignment of the spinous processes and rib angles; minor scoliosis becomes more evident when assessed in Adam's position (forward flexion in standing). Unequal distances between arms and trunk (referred to as the *keyhole*), various skin creases, or unequal muscle bulk should prompt you to closer examination. You should also assess foot and ankle alignment. Figure 7.4 provides a simple checklist for postural assessment in the clinic. View the subject from behind and assess the *symmetry* of each of the body parts shown in the first column of figure 7.4 by comparing the right and left sides of the body. Record your observations in the section headed *Notes* (e.g., "head tilted to right," "left shoulder higher than right," or "left scapula lower"). These notes will highlight the region of the body that requires local testing of muscle length and joint movement by yourself or another therapist.

Another way to assess static posture is to use a **posture grid.** The posture grid again uses a plumb line as a reference, but the subject stands behind a screen divided into 10-cm squares to aid inspection of body part alignment.

To ensure reliability of the plumb line assessment for a given client, you must perform it at the same time of day to help remove diurnal variability (Tyrrell et al. 1985). Have subjects stand with their feet 10 cm apart. They should walk on the spot (10

Table 7.1   Normal Alignment in the Sagittal Plane

Joints	Line of gravity	Gravitational torque	Opposing forces	
			Passive opposing forces	**Active opposing forces**
Atlanto-occipital	Anterior Anterior to transverse axis for flexion and extension	Flexion	Ligamentum nuchae; tectorial membrane	Posterior neck muscles
Cervical	Posterior	Extension	Anterior longitudinal ligament	
Thoracic	Anterior	Flexion	Posterior longitudinal ligament; ligamentum flavum; supraspinous ligament	Extensors
Lumbar	Posterior	Extension	Anterior longitudinal ligament	
Sacroiliac joint	Anterior	Flexion type motion	Sacrotuberous ligament; sacrospinous ligament; sacroiliac ligament	
Hip joint	Posterior	Extension	Iliofemoral ligament	Iliopsoas
Knee joint	Anterior	Extension	Posterior joint capsule	
Ankle joint	Anterior	Dorsiflexion		Soleus

Reprinted, by permission, from C.C. Norkin and P.K. Levangie, 1992, *Joint structure and function: A comprehensive analysis*, 2d ed. (Philadelphia: Davis).

paces) and then come to rest, to aid general body relaxation. Instruct your clients to maintain their "normal" posture rather than to seek to modify or improve it.

You can refine whole-body posture analysis by measuring alignment of individual body segments. You can assess pelvic tilt with a pelvic inclinometer, which measures the angle of pelvic tilt relative to the horizontal. The inclinometer consists of a protractor mounted on a base plate and attached to a pair of bone calipers. The inclinometer reads 0° when the caliper arms are horizontal. The end of the arms are positioned over the posterior superior iliac spine and the anterior superior iliac spine of one side of the body. The inclinometer dial shows the angle of pelvic tilt in the

	Position of body part	Notes
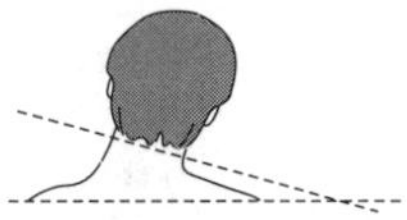	Head position	
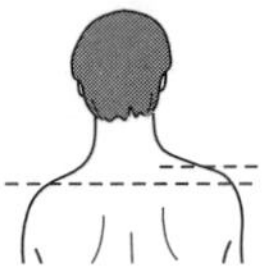	Shoulder level	
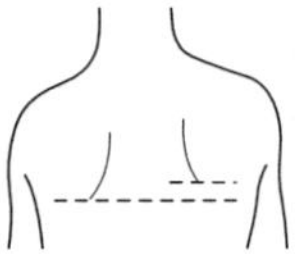	Position of shoulder blade alignment	
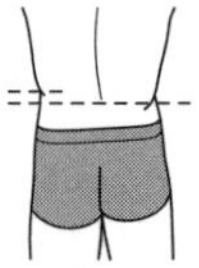	Skin creases at waist and spinal alignment	
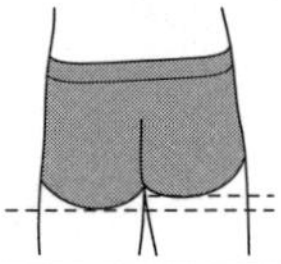	Level of buttock creases	
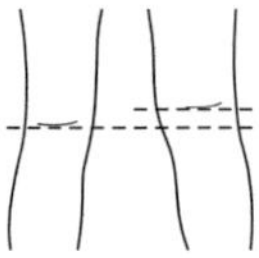	Level of knee creases	
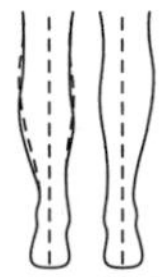	Calf muscle bulk and Achilles alignment	
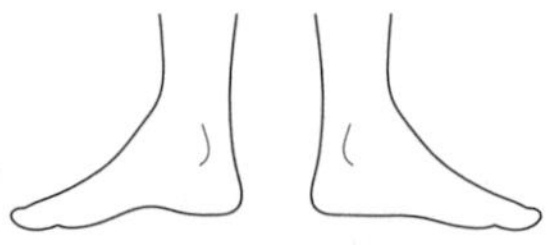	Flat foot or high arch	

Figure 7.4 Assessing standing posture from behind.

From C. Norris, 1998, *Diagnosis and management*, 2d ed. (Oxford: Butterworth Heinemann). Reprinted by permission of Butterworth Heinemann Publishers, a division of Reed Educational & Professional Publishing Ltd.

sagittal plane. This method of assessing pelvic tilt appears to be accurate to within ± ¼° (Toppenberg and Bullock 1986).

Inclinometers are highly reliable and quite valid in comparison with lateral radiographs (Crowell et al. 1994). Pelvic tilt and lumbar lordosis are intimately linked, with changes in pelvic tilt causing significant alteration in the depth of the lordosis (Day et al. 1984). Bullock-Saxton (1993) demonstrated that inclinometer measurement is repeatable in both normal and symptomatic females: subjects were measured three times on a single day with three-minute intervals between consecutive tests, and then over three separate days with a four-day rest period between each test.

You can use a flexible ruler to measure the depth of lordosis. Locate the spinous process of the second sacral segment (S2), which lies between the posterior superior iliac spines. Palpate each spinous process from S2, counting back to the first lumbar vertebra (L1) (figure 7.5). Record the length

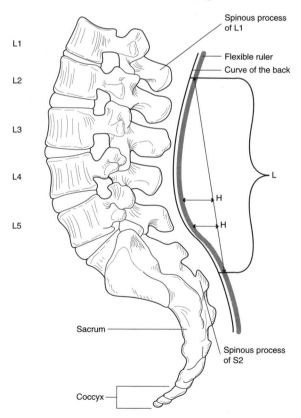

Figure 7.5 S2 lies between the posterior superior iliac spines. Palpate each spinous process cephalically from S2 up to L1. Use a flexible ruler to assess the depth of lumbar lordosis.

(radius) of the traced curvature (L) of the lordosis from L1 to S2 and the depth of the lordosis (H) from the line joining L1-S2 to the deepest part of the lordotic curve, as shown on figure 7.5. Calculate the **lordotic index** (Θ) using the **arctan formula,**

$$\Theta = 4 \arctan(2H/L).$$

Arctan is a trigonometric term that can be calculated on most scientific calculators or computer spreadsheet programs. The flexible ruler method of assessing lordosis is highly reliable, as verified by lateral radiographs (Hart and Rose 1986; Lovell et al. 1989). Lordosis measured in this manner showed average (mean) values of 50.9° in normal individuals and 40.4° in subjects who demonstrated lower abdominal weakness, confirmed as an inability to maintain alignment on supine leg lowering tasks (Levine et al. 1997).

Detect head position relative to trunk position with a stadiometer, an apparatus used to measure horizontal displacement of body segments relative to each other. The stadiometer consists of two or more sliding arms mounted on a vertical frame. The arms may be raised or lowered to the level of the body segments being measured, and then adjusted forward and backward (horizontally). A scale on the side of the horizontal arm shows the distance of each body segment from the vertical arm. Record the craniovertebral (CV) angle by measuring the degree of forward shift of the head, which pulls the suboccipital region into hyperextension (Watson 1994). The CV angle is that formed between a horizontal line through the C7 spinous process and the tragus (the prominence on the inner side of the ear) (figure 7.6). The average CV angle in asymptomatic subjects is 50° (range 48.6-52.0°); people who complain of cervical headaches have reduced angles (44.3°) (Watson 1994), indicating a head-held-forward posture as described by McKenzie (1990).

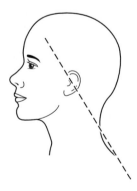

Figure 7.6 Using a stadiometer to measure the craniovertebral (CV) angle.

KEY POINT: Local "low-tech" measures of posture can be valid, reliable, and reproducible.

PRINCIPLES OF POSTURAL CORRECTION

Correcting posture requires a combination of several factors, embracing the approach to muscle imbalance described in chapter 5. Shortened muscles must be stretched, and lengthened muscle shortened. Static and PNF techniques can stretch muscles, while inner-range holding techniques can shorten lengthened muscles and build postural holding time. You must use principles of motor skill training (Norris 1998).

Make use of the three stages of motor skill training to help your clients regain segmental control (table 7.2). In the cognitive stage, your client must learn objectively the requirements of a skill. In terms of postural re-education, this often involves passive positioning of optimal posture—you place your clients passively into the optimal postural alignment by correcting pelvic tilt, for example, and instruct them to hold this position. This passive positioning is repeated several times until your clients are able to recreate the optimal position themselves. This signifies that they have progressed to the second stage of skill training (motor). During the second stage, the key factor is that individuals can identify their own mistakes. In the case of posture this means that they can consciously move into the optimal posture. Once they have achieved this ability, they are ready to perform a home-exercise program designed to build endurance

Table 7.2 Stages of Motor Skill Learning

Cognitive	Motor	Automatic
▪ Stage of understanding	▪ Effective movement now obtained	▪ Movement "runs by itself"
▪ Environmental cues important	▪ Movement more consistent	▪ Independent of attention demands
▪ Use information from past experiences	▪ Able to identify own mistakes	▪ Action very fast
▪ Poorly coordinated	▪ Proprioception more important than visual	
▪ Unable to identify own mistakes		
▪ Visual/verbal cues more important than proprioceptive		
▪ Much coaching needed		

of the postural muscles. Only after many thousands of repetitions of a movement will a person move into the third and final stage of motor training (automatic). Now, he is able to maintain an optimal postural alignment without conscious control because the action has become automatic.

The process of learning to drive a car illustrates the three stages of motor learning. When we first learn to drive, the actions are difficult and we must concentrate on many separate activities. The actions become easier with repetition, as we begin to integrate the independent actions into a whole. Eventually, driving becomes largely automatic. Similarly, the separate components of postural control must be corrected individually and then pieced together to form a more complex single movement. By dividing the total movement into a number of component sequences, you can help your client learn the action more easily.

Correcting a posture so that the correction becomes automatic is extremely difficult. If poor posture is held by shortened tissue, stretching can sufficiently lengthen tissue so that posture can change permanently—assuming that the tissue is not allowed to shorten again through poor postural alignment. If poor posture is the result of muscle weakness brought on through injury (wasting or pain inhibition), muscle strengthening may successfully optimize posture.

For many cases of poor stability, progressive exercises and proprioceptive training can effectively enhance stability and produce positive postural changes. When posture has been suboptimal for many years, however, full correction probably is not possible. Certainly improvements can be made, and these may be clinically significant (especially in relieving pain), but they will be limited.

As an example of postural re-education, consider how you might treat common lordotic posture. This posture combines lack of active lumbar stability, lengthening of the rectus abdominis, and shortening of both hamstrings and hip flexors; moreover, the gluteus maximus often is poorly recruited. Re-education begins with stabilization training for the back, emphasizing use of the deep abdominals. Once your client has enhanced her basic stability, she should stretch her hamstrings. She could then combine the two separate activities, using a hamstring stretch in sitting position while maintaining spinal alignment. Following work to improve recruitment of the gluteals, stretch the hip flexors, and shorten the rectus abdominis, she should begin whole-body postural re-education using standing, walking, and sitting movements. Finally, she would begin proprioceptive training as described on page 197.

Especially in the early stages of learning, you could use taping to give your client feedback. The taping performs two functions: First, **structural taping** or bracing can support a hypermobile segment of the body; second, **functional taping** can provide tactile feedback. In the latter case, skin drag will remind your client that her posture has moved away from the optimal alignment (place breathable undertaping under zinc oxide tape to protect the skin) (Norris 1994b).

POSTURE TYPES AND HOW TO CORRECT THEM

There are four classic abnormal posture types (figure 7.7). In the **lordotic** posture, the main feature is excessive anterior pelvic tilt (a). Anterior displacement of the pelvis characterizes the **swayback** (b), while the **flatback** has slight posterior pelvic tilting and loss of lumbar lordosis (c). In the **kyphotic** posture the thoracic curve is excessive (d).

Lordotic Posture

In the classic lordotic or "hollow back" posture, the greater trochanter remains on the LOG, but the pelvis tilts anteriorly, moving the anterior superior iliac spine (ASIS) forward and downward in relation to the pubic bone. The abdominal muscles and gluteals are typically lengthened and have poor tone. Over time, the hip flexors may shorten, and pelvic tilt is limited by tightness in the overactive and tight hamstrings (Jull and Janda 1987). In an extreme lordotic posture seen in chronic obesity, the lumbar spine rests in extension with the lumbar facet joints impacted; the elastic recoil of the hamstrings allows the pelvis to hang. Janda and Schmid (1980) call this posture the **pelvic crossed syndrome:** high contact pressures occur in the facet joints, with the inferior articular processes impinging on the lamina

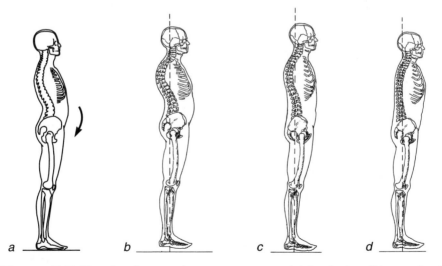

Figure 7.7 Classic abnormal posture types: *(a)* lordotic; *(b)* swayback; *(c)* flatback; and *(d)* kyphotic.

below. Increased weightbearing of the facet joints in turn reduces the compression force on the lumbar discs (Adams et al. 1994).

Lordotic posture is common in dancers and in young gymnasts, for whom it is a requirement of the sport. It is the posture most noticeable in women after childbirth, especially multiple births. In the case of childbirth, however, lengthening of the rectus abdominis through serial sarcomere adaptation is accompanied by diastasis, which may or may not resolve spontaneously.

Correction of lordotic posture requires shortening the abdominal muscles and lengthening the hip flexors. The rectus abdominis must be shortened by combining a posterior pelvic tilt with spinal flexion—but only *after* developing effective *deep* abdominal muscles to prevent bowstringing, where the abdominal muscles contract and bulge outward instead of pulling flat. This is different from the diastasis that occurs during pregnancy. With bowstringing there is no long-term structural change in the muscle, nor does the linea alba (the tendinous line between the two rectus abdominis muscles) split.

Modified Trunk Curl

GOAL *To shorten and strengthen the rectus abdominis muscle.*

The modified trunk curl action can help correct lordotic posture. Where full inner-range motion is lacking due to muscle lengthening, your client can perform the modified trunk curl in progressive stages. In stage 1, he lies supine with the knees bent and then posteriorly tilts his pelvis. Then have him curl up as far as he is able, combining spinal flexion with posterior pelvic tilt to fully shorten the rectus abdominis muscle. For stage 2, your client needs assistance either from you or from himself. You can gently pull your client into a slightly higher position, or he can pull himself higher by gripping his thighs. The extra lift should be no more than 1 or 2 inches (2.5-5.0 cm) and must be performed slowly and with care to avoid jolting the spine. Have your client hold the upper position with an isometric contraction for stage 4 (stage 3 is for those who can't perform stage 4), gradually building up the holding time from 1-2 seconds to 4-5 and finally to 10 seconds, at all times breathing normally. Individuals unable to hold the upper position should practice eccentric lowering, which represents stage 3: after they are lifted into the upper position and released, they should slow their descent back to the floor as much as possible. Initially they may almost fall back to the floor in less than 1 second. With practice, they should be able to lower themselves more slowly, taking 1-2 and then 4-5 and finally a full 10 seconds to lower

continued

Modified Trunk Curl, continued

themselves. When they have achieved this level of strength, they can progress to holding the full upper position as for stage 4.

How will you know if the abdominal muscles are lengthened and require shortening by this full inner-range holding method? In chapter 5, we saw that the length-tension curve moves to the right for lengthened muscles (see figure 5.8, page 101), indicating that they are unable to hold a joint at full inner range (i.e., to close the joint fully). When your clients perform the trunk curl, they are attempting full spinal flexion. If, in an attempt to pull the spine into full flexion, they fall back away from the inner-range position while performing the extra lift (with your help or by pulling on their thighs), you can safely conclude that the muscle is lengthened and requires this type of training to shorten it. Normally, full-range flexion of the spine is not recommended for general back care. Individuals with lordotic posture, however, have been maintaining the lumbar spine in extension. Full flexion is therefore a treatment of choice for such individuals and is widely used within physical therapy practice (McKenzie 1981).

Gluteus Maximus Inner-Range Exercise

GOAL *To contract and fully shorten the gluteus maximus.*

The gluteus maximus muscles must be tightened and shortened by working them in inner range (page 104). Have your client lie prone and flex one knee to 90°. She should then extend her hip, trying to emphasize the action of the gluteal muscles. If she is unable to lift the leg into full inner range, lift the leg for her. Then she should try either to hold this position (isometric) or to control the leg as it descends (eccentric). She eventually should attain full inner-range holding ability, with holding times built up from 3-5 seconds to 30-60 seconds.

Take a gradual, progressive approach for those who are unable to lift the leg, always remembering to adapt the program to your client's individual level of progress. Begin with muscle re-education, encouraging your client simply to contract the gluteus in prone lying. Use of EMG feedback and manual muscle stimulation is helpful at this stage if the individual is completely unable to perform a static contraction. Tapping or brushing the gluteus with the fingers adds to multisensory cueing, making the task easier by increasing the amount of information that accompanies the movement. By making the contractions forceful, your client can increase the holding time until she can contract and hold the muscle for 10 seconds. Once she can do that, the next step is to lift the

continued

Gluteus Maximus Inner-Range Exercise, continued

femur into 10-15° extension and place the knee on a block or cushion to maintain the extended hip position. She then contracts and holds the muscle as before, but in this new starting position. Eventually, she will develop sufficient strength so that you can remove the cushion and ask her to hold the extended position by herself.

If your client is unable to hold this nonsupported position, have her use eccentric lowering. After you have raised her hip into 15° extension, instruct her to hold it there as you release the leg. Encourage her to use the same intensity of muscle contraction as for the first two movements. If she is unable to hold the leg into extension (i.e., off the examination table), she should try to lower it in a controlled way rather than allowing it to drop. Have her gradually increase the time required to lower the leg to at least 10 seconds.

The next stage is for your client to forcibly contract the gluteal muscles and simultaneously try to lift the leg off the table into extension. Suggest that she bend the knee to reduce the hamstrings' contribution to extension. Begin with 2-5 repetitions, lifting the leg as high as possible without allowing the pelvis to tilt. Try placing your hand just above your client's heel on the lifting leg and then encouraging her to lift the leg until her heel touches your hand.

The final progression is first to lift the leg to full extension and hold this inner-range position for a full 10 seconds and then to perform 10 repetitions of this movement.

If clients have both poor tone in the gluteals and poor control of hip extension in the prone position, have them begin a progression of exercises leading toward the goal of performing 10 repetitions, with each contraction held 10 seconds, at each exercise session. For the first week, they should perform the exercises only every other day to reduce the likelihood of muscle soreness. They should perform 2 sets of 10 repetitions, one in the morning and one in the evening, for the first two exercise days, then 3 sets (morning, late afternoon, and evening) on the next two exercise days. Instruct clients to work gradually on increasing reps and holding time—perhaps starting with 3 repetitions, held as long as possible, then alternating between adding to the number of reps and increasing the holding time. Once they can hold a full contraction in both prone position and in extension, they should do the exercises 10 times twice per day for two days followed by 10 reps three times per day for two days. They should take a full day's rest after each four-day cycle. They should follow the sequence of 2 sets/day for two days, then 3 sets/day for two days, followed by one day of rest, for each progression until they can consistently perform 10 reps at each session, holding each rep for 10 seconds. *continued*

Gluteus Maximus Inner-Range Exercise, continued

Although this kind of inner-range exercise may shorten the previously lengthened rectus abdominis and gluteus maximus, excessive pelvic tilt will be corrected only if the tight hip flexors are stretched to release the pull on the pelvis through the iliacus muscle. Tightness of the hip flexors (*if* due to increased muscle tone rather than to adaptive shortening of connective tissue) inhibits the activity of the hip extensors through a process called *pseudoparesis* (Janda 1986). When this is the case, an individual must reduce muscle tone in the hip flexors before engaging in exercises to strengthen the hip extensors. The Thomas test (page 114) can show if the hip flexors are tight and whether the rectus femoris or iliopsoas is the tighter muscle. You also can prescribe the Thomas test for initial stretching of the hip flexors, later using the half lunge to combine lumbar stability with hip flexor stretching.

Half Lunge (without chair—see page 114)

GOAL *To stretch the hip flexors while maintaining back stability.*

Instruct your clients to assume a half-kneeling position and to tighten their abdominal muscles (using a hollowing action) to stabilize the pelvis. From this position, they should press the pelvis forward to force the trailing hip into extension. Providing the pelvis is not allowed to anteriorly tilt, the hip flexors will be stretched. Prescribe twice-daily exercise for four days, 10 repetitions per session, holding the position 20-30 seconds for each repetition. Instruct your clients to rest for a day, then repeat the four-day cycle until they have gained the desired range of motion, or until range improvement has stopped. The long-term maintenance exercise schedule should be 10 repetitions, three times per week. A chair may be useful for the client to hold (page 114) if they find the balance of this exercise difficult.

Back Flattening

GOAL *Stretches hip flexors and strengthens/builds endurance in the abdominal muscles, while re-educating posture control.*

Once an individual has corrected the muscle imbalance of the lordotic posture, he should practice assuming optimal posture. A back flattening exercise can help. Have your client stand with his back flat against a wall and his feet 6 inches (15 cm) from the wall. He should then tighten

continued

Back Flattening, continued

the abdominal muscles and gluteals in order to posteriorly tilt the pelvis, while his legs remain fully extended. The posterior pelvic tilting will effectively stretch the hip flexors. He can gradually increase the holding time, starting at 3-5 seconds and building to 30-60 seconds, breathing normally throughout the exercise. Prescribe exercises twice daily for 10 repetitions, with each repetition held 5 seconds, and a rest day taken after every four exercise days.

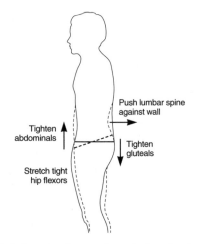

Strengthening the abdominal muscles is *not* sufficient to correct a lordotic posture. Unless a person modifies hip flexor tightness and corrects abnormal lengthening of abdominal muscles, abdominal strength changes will have little effect on pelvic tilt or lumbar lordosis. Walker et al. (1987) and Levine et al. (1997) both examined the effects of abdominal strengthening alone and found no changes in postural variables.

Swayback

In the swayback or "slouched" posture, the pelvis remains level, but the hip joint is pushed forward, the greater trochanter lying anterior to the LOG. Whereas in normal posture the sternum is the most anterior structure, now the pelvis has shifted and become the more anterior body segment, with the LOG moving from the ankle to the midfoot and toes (see figure 7.7b, page 145). The hip is effectively extended, lengthening the hip flexors, and the body "hangs" on the hip ligaments and anterior hip structures. The lordosis now changes shape from an even curve to a deeper, shorter curve with a prominent crease normally at L3 level. The kyphosis is now longer and may extend into the lumbar spine. The lower lumbar region is flatter than normal, and the pelvis may be minimally posteriorly tilted. A person with this posture will often be able to point to the exact point of pain, which normally occurs after prolonged standing. Swayback is common in youth and is the most common posture in young (18-28 years) athletes (Norris and Berry 1998).

The rectus abdominis remains relatively unchanged in the swayback posture because the pubic bone and lower ribs in general retain their anatomical relationship. However, due to the direction of the fibers of the oblique abdominals, the external oblique is lengthened and the internal oblique unchanged or shortened (figure 7.8); in the latter case, it is the upper fibers that are affected (Kendall et al. 1993).

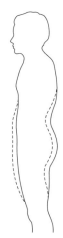

Figure 7.8 Changing length of the oblique abdominals in swayback posture.

The swayback posture may be combined with dominance of one leg in standing ("hanging on the hip"), especially in adolescents. In this case, weakness in the gluteus medius allows the pelvis to tip laterally, a situation partially compensated by increased tone in the tensor fasciae latae. Shortening is seen in the iliotibial band (ITB), with a prominent groove apparent on the lateral aspect of the thigh, as the tight fascial band pulls on the skin. You can assess tightness in the ITB using the Ober test (see page 108), which you may also use to stretch the tight muscle. Assess the ability of the gluteus medius to maintain pelvic stability in single-leg standing by using the Trendelenburg sign test (see page 73). Page 105 shows the inner-range holding test position of this muscle in side lying. Correction of swayback relies on two essential points of the posture type: the pelvis is the most anteriorly placed structure instead of the sternum, and the posture results in height loss. To correct the posture, you must help your client change the relative alignment of chest and pelvis.

Correction of Swayback Posture

GOAL *For re-education of body segment positioning.*

Have your client stand with his pelvis against the top of a table; from this position he presses his chest forward, shifting it as a single segment and avoiding any spinal flexion. At the same time, he performs abdominal hollowing to re-educate the flat abdomen alignment.

If you have observed single-leg dominance with the swayback posture, help your client correct it by stretching the adductor muscle group on the tight side, and enhancing the endurance of the abductors (gluteus medius) on the lax side. Symmetry between the two legs is essential. Use the Ober test (page 108) on both legs to determine the length of the hip abductors.

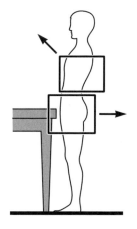

continued

Correction of Swayback Posture, continued

Determine hip adductor length by passively stretching your client's straightened leg into an abducted position, with a total of 90° hip abduction (45° on each leg) being desirable.

You can use the following two exercises both to assess the range of hip abduction and to develop it. The first assesses tightness in only the short adductors inserting above the knee (adductor longus, adductor brevis, adductor magnus) because the knee is allowed to bend. The second targets the long adductor inserting below the knee (gracilis) by keeping the knee straight throughout the stretch.

Sitting Bilateral Hip Adductor Stretch

GOAL *To stretch the hip adductors, excluding the gracilis.*

Have your client sit on the floor on a folded towel (2 inches thick), her back supported against a wall. She should place the soles of her feet together, grip the feet, and press down on her knees using her elbows, holding the full stretch for 5-10 seconds while maintaining back alignment. A desirable range of motion is for the knees to fall to within 3-4 inches of the floor. Prescribe 10 repetitions daily.

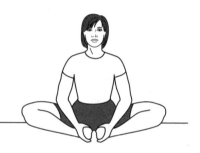

Sitting Wide Splits

GOAL *To stretch all the hip adductor muscles.*

Have your client sit on the floor in an upright posture with her arms behind her, hands on the floor to stop her from leaning back too far, legs straight. The body should be as vertical as possible. Instruct her to abduct her legs as far as possible, allowing the pelvis to posteriorly tilt. This posterior tilt will take the stretch off the adductors slightly, enabling the subject to get into the position comfortably. Then, she can increase the stretch by maintaining the position of the feet and pressing the hands against the floor to lengthen the trunk (the instructor can use the instruction "grow taller" or "try to reach your head up to

continued

Sitting Wide Splits, continued

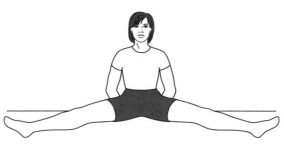

the ceiling"). As this occurs, the subject attempts to anteriorly tilt the pelvis which will move the pubic bone (the upper insertion of the adductor muscles) backwards and so increase the stretch. A desirable range of motion is a total of 90° hip abduction between both legs. She should hold the full stretch for 5-10 seconds. Prescribe 10 repetitions daily.

Because swayback posture is common in youth, but not associated with marked muscle tightening or weakening, it is difficult to correct. The emphasis is on re-education, with postural awareness playing an important part in the process. You can increase postural awareness by the use of proprioception during the spinal lengthening exercise below.

Spinal Lengthening

GOAL *To improve awareness of body position.*

Your client needs a partner for this exercise. As your client stands in his normal resting posture, his partner places a hand 1-2 inches (2.5-5.0 cm) above the crown of the client's head. Instruct your client to lengthen his spine (the instruction is to "grow taller"), attempting to touch his partner's hand with the top of his head. He must not look up (cervical extension) in an attempt to lengthen his neck, and must not stand on his toes!

Once he has mastered this action, he should attempt the same lengthening action without the help of a partner. The action is again to "grow taller." Placing a light book or beanbag on the head helps to give sensory feedback and can help him focus his attention on moving the top of his head upward. Initially he practices simple lengthening at whatever speed is comfortable, with the beanbag on the head. Eventually he should slow the lengthening action, attempting to hold the lengthened position for 5-10 seconds while breathing normally (some people take a deep breath and hold it—this must not be allowed, as it can lead to lightheadedness). The lengthened position should be relatively relaxed and not stiff—comparisons with a puppet rather than a wooden stick can illustrate the difference between stability (spine lengthened and

continued

Spinal Lengthening, continued

aligned) and rigidity (spine fixed). When your client is able to perform the movement and hold the corrected body position, he can progress to walking while holding the lengthened position, and then to simple activities such as sitting/standing from a chair to increase the variety of movements.

In order to provide sensory feedback when the swayback posture is incorrectly stretching the muscle, try applying *nonelastic* tape on the skin over the external oblique, taking up any skin slack. Attach the tape to the lower lateral aspect of the abdomen, out toward the anterior rim of the pelvis. Pull the tape tight from this point up to the posterolateral aspect of the lower ribs. Although the tape is not strong enough to prevent the pelvis from moving forward in relation to the rib cage, it will remind your client when this is happening and encourage him to correct the posture. The more times he makes the correction, the more likely it is that optimal postural alignment will become automatic. 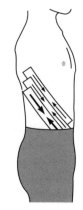 Either a physical therapist or athletic trainer should apply the tape, and it should be done immediately following the spinal lengthening exercise above, to encourage maintaining correct alignment between exercise bouts.

Another way to reinforce automatic alignment is to build correction into daily activities. Encourage your client to perform the pelvis-chest realignment exercise regularly throughout the day. Office workers, for example, can perform the exercise whenever the telephone rings, and students can perform it each time a bell rings to end class.

If the iliopsoas is lengthened by the extended position of the hip (the Thomas test will reveal this; see chapter 5) its inner-range holding must be redeveloped.

Sitting, Hip Flexor Shortening

GOAL *To shorten the iliopsoas and rectus femoris muscles and build their endurance.*

While your client is sitting, you should passively flex the hip to the maximum degree possible without pain—or to approximately 110°, or to the point where the pelvis just begins to posteriorly rotate. Instruct your client to hold this position for 10 seconds, while maintaining a

continued

Sitting, Hip Flexor Shortening, continued

neutral lordosis. Inability to hold at full inner range for 10 repetitions (10 seconds each) is a sign of postural lengthening. If the iliopsoas is lengthened, the leg may drop and/or the pelvis drop back into posterior tilt, moving the iliopsoas into its lengthened position. Your client can redevelop inner-range holding of the iliopsoas by using first eccentric and then isometric inner-range hip flexor exercises while maintaining a neutral lordosis.

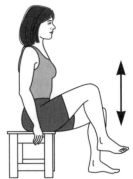

In the preceding exercise position, your client should try to lift her leg to full flexion. Then you should try to lift the leg farther (increasing hip flexion), *without* altering the position of the spine or pelvis. Remember that a lengthened muscle cannot contract powerfully to pull a limb into its fully closed (inner-range) position. If your client's hip flexors are lengthened, further passive movement will be possible because she will not have been able to pull her own leg into full inner range. Have her attempt to hold this new (passive) inner-range position. If she is able to do so, instruct her to build up holding time from 1-2 seconds to 10 seconds while performing the exercise daily for two weeks—her target is 10 repetitions of the 10-second hold.

If your client is not able to hold the passive inner-range position, she should use controlled lowering (eccentric). From the passive inner-range position, she attempts to slow the descent of the leg after you release it from its fully flexed position. She should continue the controlled lowering until she can slow the descent sufficiently to hold the leg still. She then progresses to holding at reducing joint angles. For example, assume that the *active* inner-range position (with your client using her own muscles) is 90° hip flexion, and the *passive* inner-range position (as you lift the leg farther into flexion) is 120°. The target for active flexion/holding is about 110°. You lift her leg to 120° hip flexion and release the leg. She then controls the lowering back to the 90° starting position. Once she can do this consistently, you lift her leg to 90-100° and she attempts to hold it. Once she can hold this position, you repeat the exercise, beginning again with the 110-120° passive flexion.

She should perform each holding or lowering exercise only five times before taking a rest period since the muscle fatigues quickly with this exercise and alignment will be lost. Prescribe 3 sets of 5 repetitions twice daily for four days (a family member can provide the passive flexion), followed by a single day of rest, then another five-day cycle, and so on. The goal is the ability to actively flex the leg to 110° and hold it for 10 seconds for each exercise set.

Flatback

With the flatback posture, the main problem is lack of mobility in the lumbar spine and a flattening of the lordosis (lumbar flexion). This posture reflects the extension dysfunction described by McKenzie (1981) and is common in chronic low back pain after extended periods of inactivity. The pelvis may be posteriorly tilted in comparison to the reference line, and the lumbar tissues are often thickened and immobile. The flatback posture is also seen in subjects who practice a high number of sit-up type exercises (repeated lumbar flexion). In this case the lumbar spine may be mobile—but the rectus abdominis is strong and tight, and is by far the dominant member of the abdominal muscle group.

Flatback is corrected by regaining appropriate mobility in the lumbar spine through passive and active extension movements.

Passive Back Extension in Lying Position

GOAL *To improve the passive range of extension in the lumbar spine.*

Performed in the lying position, extension exercises first mobilize the upper lumbar levels, with proportionally less caudal movement (McKenzie 1981). Instruct your client to lie prone on the lab table (or floor), with his hands by his shoulders in a push-up position (a). He should extend his arms

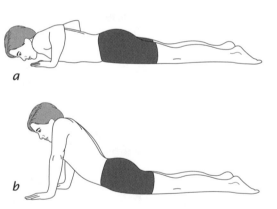

while keeping his pelvis on the table, thereby forcing extension of the spine (b). Initially, some people may need to push up only with their forearms on the table, gradually building up to full arm extension. To emphasize the motion of the spine rather than the pelvis, try fixing the pelvis to the table with a webbing belt.

If your client experiences any pain in the lumbar region during this exercise, refer him to a physical therapist (PT). Often, instead of the whole lumbar spine being stiff to extension, one or two vertebrae may be stiffer than others. These stiff units require a specific manual therapy tech-

continued

Passive Back Extension in Lying Position, continued

nique of "joint mobilization" either before or during the exercise program. When a specific stiff area has started to move (the PT will assess this), you can move the webbing belt up or down within the lumbar region to form a fulcrum around which the movement occurs. In this way, the extension action is focused more exactly on a single lumbar joint.

See that your clients practice the passive extension movement often, but for only a short time each session, to allow the movement to develop without causing too much reactionary pain. Suggest 10 repetitions every two hours throughout the waking day, with a full day's rest after every four days. The exercise should continue until the individual has achieved the desired movement range.

Pelvic Tilt Re-Education, Sitting

GOAL *To regain both range and quality of movement in the lumbar spine.*

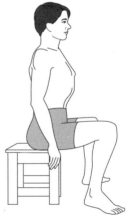

If the lower lumbar spine has reduced extension, the pelvic tilting action may be effective in correcting it. Instruct your client to sit on a low stool with his feet on the ground. Keeping his shoulders still, he should try to tilt his pelvis forward and down. Tell him to think of his pelvis as a bowl full of water, and that by tilting the bowl he can pour the water onto the ground between his feet. He should try to bring the backside of the bowl up as he pushes the front of it down, always keeping his shoulders still and his sternum up.

When the motion is especially poor, provide passive assistance. Wrap a webbing belt around your client's waist and, fixing the sternum, pull the lumbar spine into extension as he attempts to tilt his pelvis (see page 75, "Assisted Pelvic Tilting While Sitting"). Refer to chapter 4 for a fuller discussion of pelvic tilt.

Kyphotic Back

In the kyphotic posture, the shoulder joint moves anteriorly to the posture line, increasing the thoracic kyphosis. In optimal upper body alignment (table 7.3), the scapulae should be approximately the width of three fingers from the spine, and the medial borders of the scapulae should be vertical. Assess optimal positioning of the shoulder by comparing the head of the humerus in relation to the acromion process. In optimal positioning, no more that one-third of the humeral head should be anterior to the point of the acromion. The humerus should be held with the cubital fossa (elbow crease) at 45° to the sagittal plane in relaxed standing. A smaller angle indicates excessive medial rotation, indicating tightness in the medial rotators (especially the pectoralis major) and lengthening of the lateral rotators. Visualizing how this would appear from above may be helpful. When the arm is held in medial rotation, the crease of the elbow is orientated more forward and inward; when lateral rotation is greater than normal, the elbow crease faces farther outward.

Deviation from the ideal is often described as a "round-shouldered" posture, a blanket term that covers a number of scenarios. Tightness in the anterior structures pulls the shoulder forward, away from the posture line. The weight of the arm moves farther from the upper body's center of gravity, dramatically increasing the leverage forces transmitted to the thorax. Eventually, thoracic kyphosis increases. Tightness in the pectoralis minor pulls on the coracoid process, tilting the scapula forward (figure 7.9a). Tightness in the pectoralis major causes both excessive medial rotation at the glenohumeral joint and anterior displacement of the humeral head (figure 7.9b). Lengthening of the lower trapezius and serratus anterior may cause excessive abduction (figure 7.9c) and downward rotation (figure 7.9d) of the scapula. Excessive elevation (figure 7.9e) and upward rotation may result from tightness in the upper fibers of the trapezius.

Correction of kyphotic posture depends on flexibility of the thoracic spine. Where the kyphosis appears *fixed* and thoracic motion is grossly reduced, thoracic joint mobilization is required as a first step. Once some mobility has been gained passively by manual therapy, you can use exer-

Table 7.3 Correct Alignment of the Shoulder Girdle

From behind	From the side
• Medial border of scapula vertical	• Line from ear canal to center of shoulder joint is perpendicular to floor
• Medial border of scapula no more than three finger breadths from the spinous processes	• No more than one-third of head of humerus anterior to acromion
• Spine of scapular T3/T4 level, inferior angle at T7	• Humerus held with elbow crease 45° to sagittal plane
• Scapula flat against thoracic wall	

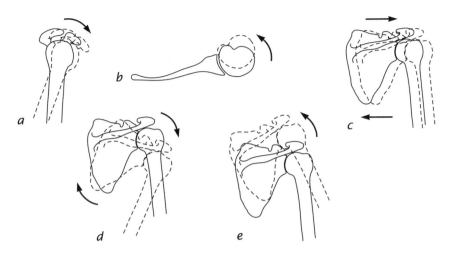

Figure 7.9 Postural changes around the shoulder.

cise therapy to maintain the newly gained motion. The sternal lift action (page 162) is the exercise of choice. If the subject is younger and the thoracic spine is *mobile*, only scapular repositioning is required.

Thoracic Joint Mobilization

GOAL *To increase mobility of thoracic joints, using manual therapy, in preparation for exercise therapy.*

With your client in the prone lying position, work with a PT to use posterior-anterior vertebral pressures (PAVP) or gross extension pressures to isolate the thoracic spine. With your client sitting, you can combine mobilization with overpressure. Have her sit facing a treatment table, with her arms folded and placed on the table. As you press the thoracic spine into extension, instruct her to try to follow the action. If thoracic mobility is quite limited, at first you will simply press the spine passively into extension. As your client gains mobility, encourage her to follow your motion with her own active movement while you gradually reduce the pressure you apply. The first step in this active process is for the subject to be able to "feel" the movement. Many people with a kyphotic posture have a poor ability to control the quality of motion in the thoracic spine, and this type of guided exercise can help them improve their control. If your client is still unable to perform active thoracic extension even after regaining passive extension, suggest a visualization technique: encourage her to *imagine* herself performing the action.

continued

Thoracic Joint Mobilization, continued

Either you or a model should perform the action correctly. You can also use video to enable your client to see the action from behind, while a mirror provides a view from the front. Then have her repeat her attempt at active thoracic extension. She may need to cycle through a series of visualization sessions, passive extension, and attempts at active extension before she can finally sense what active extension feels like. Once that happens, she can proceed to daily exercises. The subject should perform the exercise daily for 10-15 repetitions. In the early 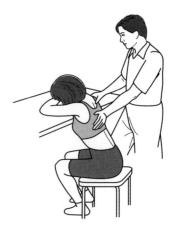 stages as mobility is very poor, some soreness can be expected following the exercise, so a greater number of repetitions should not be performed.

Scapula Repositioning

GOAL *To improve control of scapular retraction and depression.*

If the thoracic spine is mobile, you can correct kyphotic posture by repositioning the scapulae—shortening the shoulder retractors and enhancing the scapular stabilizers (especially lower trapezius and serratus anterior). The aim here is to improve control of movement rather than simply to increase strength. By improving strength, muscle endurance, and movement quality (coordination and timing), these exercises differ from many traditional weight-training programs whose primary aims are gains in strength and muscle size.

With your client lying prone, passively place his scapula into optimal alignment—the medial borders vertical, three finger widths from the spine. The scapula should be firmly anchored to the thorax (by action of the serratus anterior and lower trapezius muscles) rather than being separated from the rib cage. Frequently this involves passively depressing and adducting the scapula, but the amount of passive movement of the scapula that is required depends on the postural alignment of the subject. More movement is needed in subjects who have grossly abducted scapulae (medial border of scapula 5-6 inches [13-15 cm] from the spine) than for those with minimal abduction (medial border 3-4 inches [8-10 cm] from the spine) (Mottram 1997; Norris 1998).

Initially, encourage your client to hold the new position for 1-2 seconds. Often the tendency is for the subject to "brace" the shoulders back

continued

Scapula Repositioning, continued

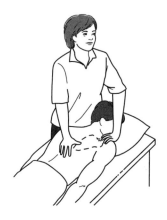

hard. Discourage this reaction since it requires maximal muscle activity. Encourage your client to "let go" until the scapula just begins to move away from the corrected position, and then to hold the muscles slightly tight. Progressively increase the amount of time that this position is held with minimal muscle work, from 1-2 to 3-4 and eventually 10 seconds. The aim is to build up to 10 reps, holding each for 10 seconds, with the minimal amount of scapular muscle work that is required to maintain good scapular alignment.

Tight anterior structures must be stretched to allow the shoulders to retract fully. Check for tightness in the pectoralis major and pectoralis minor, and if necessary prescribe stretching exercises as detailed in the following sections.

Door Frame Stretch

GOAL *Stretch pectoralis major muscles.*

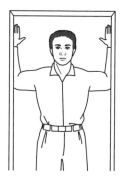

Instruct your client to lean forward onto a doorframe, his arms horizontal, his forearms vertical against the frame. He then pushes his arms back into extension by leaning into the doorway opening, holding the position for 20 seconds. Have your client do this exercise 3 times a day, with 2 repetitions each time.

Weight Bag Passive Stretch

GOAL *Stretch pectoralis minor muscles.*

A tight pectoralis minor can pull the scapula down and forward. Have your client lie in a supine position. Place a 3- to 5-lb weight bag over the anterior aspect of her shoulder. She should relax and allow the bag to press the shoulder back into position for 30 seconds. The weight bag

continued

Weight Bag Passive Stretch, continued

will help press the shoulder back into retraction, passively stretching the anterior structures. To use a contract-relax technique, the client presses the shoulder into protraction for 2 seconds, trying to lift the weight bag, and then relaxes for 5-10 seconds, allowing the weight bag to press the shoulder farther back. A static stretch may also be used with the client simply lying relaxed, allowing the weight bag to press her shoulders back.

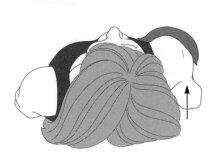

Sternal Lift Exercise

GOAL *Combines thoracic extension and scapular repositioning.*

While sitting, your client should lift his sternum using thoracic extension (rather than simply taking a deep breath) (a). At the same time, he should draw the scapulae down and in toward their optimal alignment. He may prefer to perform the action against a wall, where the movement should be one of "rolling" the thoracic spine up the wall while keeping the lumbar spine stable and avoiding any increase in the depth of the lumbar lordosis (b).

If the client's lumbar spine stability is particularly poor and he is unable to avoid hyperflexion, modify the starting position by having him sit on a bench, with his feet on a chair to bring the femur above the horizontal. This position posteriorly tilts the pelvis and flattens or reverses the lumbar lordosis.

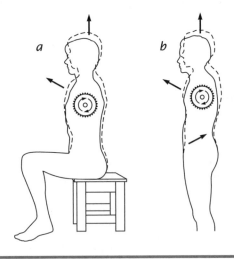

SUMMARY

- Posture is the arrangement of body parts in a state of balance that protects the supporting structures of the body against injury or progressive deformity.
- Postural sway consists of a small continuous motion in the sagittal plane—an oscillation of the center of gravity that may reduce lower-limb fatigue and aid blood flow.
- Excessive postural sway generally reveals poor balance and stability.
- You can assess clients' postures by use of a plumb line or a posture grid.
- There are four basic types of abnormal posture:
  1. Lordotic posture is characterized by excessive anterior pelvic tilt.
  2. Swayback is characterized by anterior displacement of the pelvis.
  3. Flatback is characterized by slight posterior pelvic tilting and loss of lumbar lordosis.
  4. Kyphosis is characterized by excessive thoracic curve.
- This chapter describes how to assess different abnormal posture types and presents exercises that can help correct them.

III

Building
Back Fitness

If you bring a client all the way through the assessments and exercises in the previous chapters, he or she should have a basically stable back, with no pain. Some clients need more, however—namely, those whose demands in the workplace or in sport activities require extraordinary strength, speed, or accuracy of movement.

Chapter 8 ("Advanced Stability Training") presents exercises that will build on the training already achieved, using body movements alone, using balance boards, using stability balls, or employing proprioceptive training to increase accuracy of muscle control. Chapter 9 ("More Advanced Stability Training: Weight Training and Plyometrics") is for those clients who need the most rigorous training possible for their backs because of extremely heavy sport/workplace demands. Please note: the approaches used in chapters 8 and 9 are specifically for people who have had lower-back problems and/or who need to prevent such problems in the future. Study the chapters with that in mind—the material does NOT merely re-state what you've read before about weight training, etc. Because these chapters approach advanced training from the viewpoint of increasing your client's back stability, and not simply with the idea of building pretty muscles or increasing overall strength, they will be invaluable to your clients who have major concerns about their backs.

8

Advanced Stability Training

After your clients have used the procedures and exercises of previous chapters to achieve basic back stability, they are ready (if they wish) to build on that stability. By now they should have learned to control pelvic tilt; to automatically assume the neutral position; to maintain abdominal hollowing (at 30-40% of the maximum effort); and to contract the multifidus at will—or, in quantitative terms, to perform the basic procedures in chapter 4 with variable intensity for 10 repetitions, holding each repetition for 10 seconds. With your help, they should have begun correcting muscle imbalances using the approaches in chapter 5. They should have developed their abdominal strength using the exercises in chapter 6. They should be able to maintain proper posture as described in chapter 7. Many people—who are relatively sedentary and whose back stability is rarely challenged through workplace or leisure-time activities—may have little motivation to proceed with additional training. Others will want to go further, however, especially if they are involved in sports or if they face heavy physical demands on the job. In this chapter, I cover exercises for developing even greater back stability. Chapter 9 goes further still, but your clients should master the material in this chapter before moving to the very strenuous work in that chapter.

The first class of exercises in this chapter simply adds layers of complexity onto movements your clients will already know from other chapters. But there is also an entire series of exercises using a stability ball (or "gym ball"), which was introduced briefly in chapter 4—many people find these exercises more "user friendly" for their home workouts. Finally, I cover a small core of proprioceptive exercises—training that is advanced beyond what your clients have seen thus far, and that provides a kind of transition between some of the later exercises in the first section and the plyometric exercises in chapter 9.

Very important: for each of the exercises in this chapter, your clients should gently contract their deep abdominal muscles to perform abdominal hollowing and maintain this contraction throughout the exercise. By now, moreover, they should be able to voluntarily contract the multifidus muscles—especially if they began the program as sufferers from *chronic* low back pain. They should begin all exercises in the neutral position.

SUPERIMPOSED LIMB MOVEMENTS AND BALANCE BOARDS

Each of the following exercises involves limb movements that are superimposed on a basically stable back that the exercises of chapter 4 can create (i.e., in these exercises an individual tightens the back stability muscles and then moves the limbs upon the stable base). As your clients focus their attention on limb movements, they will become more able to control their back stability muscles without conscious thought. This kind of automatic response occurs only with long repetition of the exercises. You should find it surprisingly easy to observe the point at which your clients are exerting automatic control. If they perform a limb-loading exercise such as the standing single-leg raise or the crook lying heel slide, for example, movement of the pelvis will reveal lack of back stability. In this case, you would retreat a couple of steps and have your clients practice the hollowing actions to enhance their ability to stabilize the spine. Once they have built up endurance of these muscles and can hold the abdominal contraction for 10 repetitions of 10 seconds each, you would once again try adding limb movements to the basic exercises. If they can now successfully control limb movements while avoiding unwanted pelvic movement (maintaining the lumbar spine's neutral position throughout the action), you will know that they are gaining automatic control of the stabilizing muscles—they no longer have to focus their attention on these muscles and can now concentrate on accurate positioning of the limb.

For each of the following exercises, your client should progress in a single session only to the point at which he can no longer maintain neutral position, correct pelvic tilt, or maintain abdominal hollowing. Have him do the exercise daily for four days, rest one day, then resume the pattern, gradually increasing the progression or the number of repetitions until he eventually can do the exercise in its most challenging form for 10 reps, holding (where appropriate) for 10 seconds each time. Obviously, all one-sided movements should be performed on both right and left sides, one being the mirror image of the other. Each exercise should be performed in a slow, controlled fashion, maintaining the neutral position of the spine throughout the exercise. Since limb leverage changes when arms/legs are bent and straightened, your clients will necessarily have to vary the amount of abdominal work they use to maintain the neutral position. It is this variation that makes the difference (in terms of skill) between the holding exercises, such as abdominal hollowing, and these more advanced exercises that involve limb movements upon the stable trunk base.

Determining the Starting Position

An individual's starting position depends on his physical characteristics and abilities. You should always be open, moreover, to changing the starting position if you perceive that your first choice may not have been the best—which will be the case if your client is not succeeding with an exercise. Some exercises are easier than others because they involve less muscle work. For example, in the heel slide movement, the ground partially takes the weight of the leg, while in the single-leg raise, the subject lifts the whole of the leg weight. The former exercise is therefore easier in terms of pure muscle work. Some movements may be more comfortable for certain subjects. Since lying positions are more supported than kneeling, for example, many people feel more secure in lying.

The program generally follows a neurodevelopmental progression (i.e., the sequence that children go through when they learn to sit, stand, and walk). In the present case, we go from ground support, to apparatus support, and finally to increasingly complex free exercises.

Exercises in the Crook Lying Position

The crook lying position, which was used to perform abdominal hollowing and pelvic tilting, is a good starting position for superimposed limb movements. As an individual straightens the leg or lowers it to the ground, the overload placed on the trunk becomes progressively greater—the individual must therefore vary the intensity of muscular stabilization to maintain the neutral position. This variation in muscle contraction intensity increases the person's *control* rather than simply strength or endurance capacity.

Heel Slide—the Basic Movement

GOAL *To place minimal, but progressive, limb loading on the trunk.*

Instruct your client to slowly straighten one leg, with the heel resting on the ground. This movement is easier if the heel is on a slippery surface (a cloth if on a polished floor, or a piece of shiny paper if on carpet). The moment the pelvis anteriorly tilts and the lordosis increases, the movement must stop and the leg be drawn back into flexion once more.

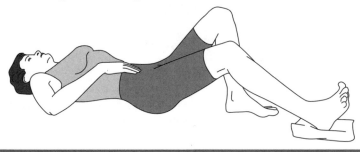

Leg Lowering

GOAL *Limb loading as a progression from the heel slide.*

Instruct your client to flex both her hips to 90° so that her thighs are vertical to the ground, while keeping her knees relaxed. She should then slowly extend one hip until her foot touches the ground. Have her gradually extend the knee farther in subsequent repetitions, so that the foot touches the ground farther from the buttock, increasing the limb leverage and therefore progressing the resistance. The exercise is performed daily for four days and then a single day's rest is taken. She should continue this sequence until she can perform the exercise with the leg almost straight. Once she can perform the exercise with the leg almost straight, she can progress to single-leg raises.

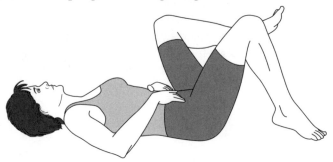

Single Bent-Leg Raises

GOAL *Progression from leg lowering.*

Beginning in the crook lying position, your client should lift one leg—still bent at the knee—while the other rests on the floor. He brings the knee up as far as he can without moving out of neutral position, then lowers it. Then he repeats with the other leg. As a progression on this action, have him begin lifting one leg just before the other limb has touched the ground so that momentarily they are both off the floor at the same time. Finally, he should lift and lower both legs together, initially with minimal limb leverage (i.e., with knees well bent) and finally with increasing leverage (legs increasingly straightened). The maximum leverage will vary with each individual. For most well-conditioned individuals, 90-120° knee extension is appropriate. At no time should the pelvis anteriorly tilt, and at no time should the abdominal muscles be allowed to bowstring (bulge outward rather than maintain a flat or hollow contour). I do *not* recommend progressing all the way to bilateral straight-leg raises—the compression and shear forces imposed by the psoas muscle upon the lumbar spine make this unsuitable for use in rehabilitation following low back pain.

KEY POINT: ▶ The neutral position of the lumbar spine must be maintained throughout the exercises. If the pelvis tilts and neutral position is lost, the exercise must be stopped, and the client should revert to an earlier stage of the exercise in which the pelvic tilt was accurately controlled. Be certain also that your clients keep their abdomens hollowed throughout the exercises.

Prone Lying Gluteal Brace

GOAL *Co-contraction of trunk stabilizers with gluteals.*

Instruct your client to lie prone, then to dorsiflex one foot, with the toes bent up toward the knee. She should then slightly flex both her knee (about 10°) and her hip (also about 10°). She then contracts her gluteal muscles to lift the femur into extension to the horizontal position (with the foot remaining on the ground), straightening the knee.

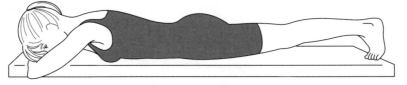

Prone Bent-Leg Lift

GOAL *Active movement of an unsupported leg on the stable trunk.*

In the prone lying position, your client should flex one leg to 90° at the knee. Instruct your client to set her abdominal muscles and contract the gluteals to lift the leg from the floor. To prevent passive anterior pelvic tilt, the maximum hip extension should be only 15°. This position places the hamstring muscles at a mechanical disadvantage, reducing the tension they can create and therefore throwing greater stress onto the gluteals. To increase the isolation of the gluteals from the hamstrings, have your client slowly flex her knee while maintaining hip extension—this causes the gluteals to act isometrically as hip stabilizers while the hamstrings acts isotonically as prime knee flexors.

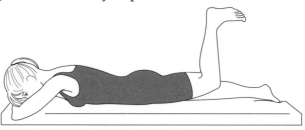

Bridge From Crook Lying

GOAL *Using leg power to lift the trunk while maintaining a neutral lumbar position.*

In a crook lying position, your client should tighten his gluteal muscles and then lift his pelvis from the ground, aiming to form a straight line from shoulders to hips and then to the knees.

This exercise tends to induce movement in the sagittal plane (anterior-posterior pelvic tilt, and/or lumbar flexion-extension). Lifting one leg (see next exercise) imposes an additional rotary stress, tending to cause movement within the transverse plane.

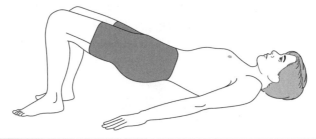

Bridge With Leg Lift

GOAL *A progression from bridge from crook lying.*

Instruct your client to assume the bridge position, starting from crook lying. Then he lifts one leg, avoiding the tendency for the pelvis to fall toward the unsupported side. Placing a stick across the anterior superior iliac spines of the pelvis gives useful feedback for keeping the pelvis level.

Exercises in 4-Point Kneeling Position

The 4-point kneeling position is initially stable since four symmetrical points (both hands and both knees) bear the weight. As one arm or one leg is lifted to reduce support to three points, the body is less stable and the stability muscles must now work harder to maintain trunk alignment and stop the body from tipping.

Four-Point Body Sway

GOAL *Learning to maintain neutral position as the limbs are moved.*

Instruct your client, who begins in the standard 4-point position, to sway the body forward and back, moving at the shoulders and hips only. As she passes the critical point of 90° hip flexion, be sure that her lumbar spine remains in its neutral position. As soon as she begins to lose the neutral lumbar position, she should reverse the movement back into full 4-point kneeling. The aim is to gradually work farther and farther back (increasing hip flexion) while maintaining a neutral spine.

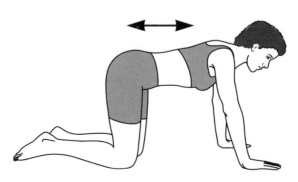

Four-Point Pelvic Shift

GOAL *Learning to unload the limbs prior to lifting them.*

After assuming the 4-point posi- tion, your client should shift to the side to take the weight of the far leg. She then barely lifts the leg on this side from the supporting surface, leaving only one knee in contact with the ground. Be sure that she lifts the leg a *maximum* of 1-2 inches 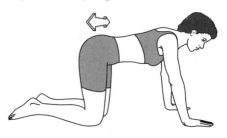 (2.5-5.0 cm). Some people find the subtlety of this movement difficult and tend to lift the leg by 6-8 inches (15-20 cm)—but this imposes an unwanted rotation on the spine and must be discouraged. Placing a stick across the upper pelvis (level with the posterior superior iliac spines) is helpful. With the required subtle movement, the stick will stay in place. If the leg is lifted too far, however, pelvic rotation will cause the stick to fall.

Four-Point Leg Flexion/Extension

GOAL *Controlling back stability in the presence of limb move- ment.*

Your client should begin as for the previous exercise, shifting weight to one leg. Instruct him to move the unloaded leg into flexion/extension and abduction/adduction, while maintaining a neutral lumbar spine and keeping the lower leg parallel to the floor. He should use only small movements, the knee moving forward/backward and side to side by only 2-3 inches (5-8 cm). Larger movements will require greater changes in pelvic tilt and are more difficult to control. The movements should be slow to avoid excessive limb momentum—no more than 1 or 2 com- plete limb movements per second.

Four-Point Kneeling Leg Lift

GOAL *Maintaining stability during increasing complexities of leg movement.*

From the basic 4-point kneeling position, your client should extend one leg completely, keeping the foot on the ground (a). The next step is to lift the leg until it is parallel to the floor (b). Finally, instruct him to alter- nately flex and extend the raised leg at the knee, keeping the raised thigh

continued

Four-Point Kneeling Leg Lift, continued

parallel to the floor. The foot should remain in a middle (neutral) position, toes and foot neither fully pointed (plantarflexed) nor fully pulled up (dorsiflexed)—holding the shin or calf muscles tight can cause muscle cramping.

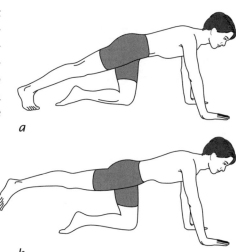

a

b

Several alignment faults are common in this final movement. First, while your client is focusing on the limb movement, he may forget to maintain contraction of the trunk stabilizing muscles—leading the abdominal wall to bulge because the hollowing action is lost. As this happens, the pelvis may anteriorly tilt, pulling the lumbar spine into excessive extension (back hollowing). Finally, if the gluteals have poor endurance, the client may start to rely on his hamstrings to maintain the extended hip position: as the hamstrings begin to flex the knee, he loses the hip extension position and the leg drops below the horizontal. In each case, you should stop the procedure and return to the previous exercise.

Four-Point Kneeling Arm and Leg Lift

GOAL *Increasing the complexity of limb movements while maintaining back stability.*

Have your client begin as with the kneeling leg lift above. But this time, once the leg reaches the horizontal, he should also lift the diagonally opposite arm. Watch to see that his shoulder does not sag or drop down on this side; the scapula should not move as the elbow bends to unload the arm. Once your client's hand has cleared the ground, he should lift the arm forward toward the horizontal.

Exercises in the Side Lying Position

We saw in chapter 7 that, in the frontal plane, the gluteus medius may lack endurance and inner-range holding ability, leading both the tensor fasciae lata/iliotibial band (TFL/ITB) and the hip adductors to tighten. In the side lying position, we are attempting to work the gluteus medius and to stretch the adductors, while maintaining stability of the pelvis and lumbar spine in the frontal plane. The stability is achieved by contraction of the lateral abdominals and the quadratus lumborum *acting together*. Where lateral abdominal function is poor, the quadratus lumborum can become overactive and tight. Each of the following exercises overloads the quadratus lumborum and the oblique abdominal muscles on the upper side of the body. The movements must be reversed to provide a symmetrical overload.

Side Lying Knee Lift

GOAL *Maintaining trunk stability in the frontal (side flexion) plane during limb movement.*

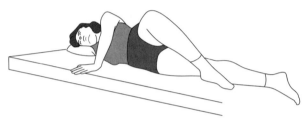

Have your client begin the exercise in side lying, and align her pelvis so that the line joining the two anterior superior iliac spines is vertical. She must maintain this alignment throughout the exercise. Do not allow lateral movement of the pelvis. Instruct her to place the foot of her top leg on the floor in front of the shin of her lower leg. Then she should lift the top knee by abducting and externally rotating her hip, keeping the foot in place on the ground. Palpate the posterior fibers of gluteus medius above and behind the greater trochanter to make sure they are contracting. Give your client feedback until she is able to tell when she is contracting these fibers as she lifts her knee. Once she is able to feel the appropriate contraction, have her attempt to lift to full inner range, but stop her immediately if the pelvis begins to move out of alignment.

Side Lying Leg Rotation

GOAL *Maintaining trunk stability and isolating pelvic control from hip rotation.*

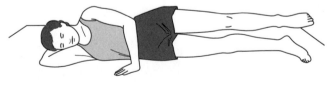

The second exercise combines abduction ability and trunk stability, while isolating hip movement from that of the pelvis. From the stabilized side lying position, your client should hold her upper leg straight and abduct it to the horizontal.

continued

Side Lying Leg Rotation, continued

Tell her to then externally rotate the entire leg from the hip, turning the foot toward the ceiling and then back to pointing forward. Have your client perform 3-5 rotations before lowering the leg, unless she loses alignment of the pelvis—in which case she should lower her leg immediately.

Side Lying Leg Abduction

GOAL *Controlling hip abduction on a stable trunk.*

The third exercise represents true abduction upon a stable base. Have your client assume the stable side lying position, then lift his upper leg into abduction while avoiding 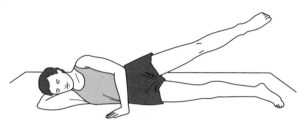 flexion and external rotation. Encourage him to "lengthen his leg" to avoid lateral pelvic movement, and then to abduct his leg as high as he can without experiencing discomfort, up to a maximum of 45° from the horizontal. All the movement should be in the hip—tell him to avoid lumbar-pelvic movement. He may have to work up gradually to the 45-degree target.

Side Lying Spine Lengthening

GOAL *Controlling the quadratus lumborum and lateral fibers of the oblique abdominals.*

Side lying is also a useful starting position for strong co-contraction of the abdominal muscles with minimal compressive and shear forces on the lumbar spine (McGill 1997). Have your client lie on his left side, his thighs in line with his body but his knees flexed 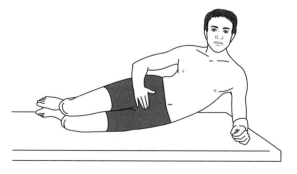 90°, with his upper body supported on his left elbow to side flex the spine. He should then straighten his spine against the force of gravity, leaving the body supported on the forearm of the underneath arm and hip.

Side Lying Hip Lift

GOAL *Progression from side lying spine lengthening.*

Have your client assume the position for the side lying spine lengthening. Then have him lift his hips, leaving the body supported on the forearm of the underneath arm and the knees.

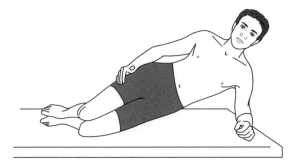

Side Lying Body Lift

GOAL *Final progression for developing control of quadratus lumborum and lateral fibers of oblique abdominals.*

Again, have your client assume the position for the side lying spine lengthening. Instruct him to straighten his knees and cross the upper leg in front of the lower leg. Then he should lift his body to the full side support position, leaving the body supported on the forearm of the underneath arm and the feet. Encourage him to "lengthen his body" and to "broaden his shoulders" to avoid their "falling" into scapular adduction—the aim being to form a straight line from the feet, through the pelvis, to the shoulders.

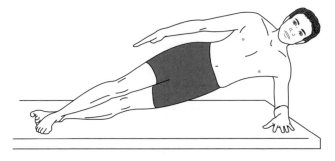

Exercises in the Standing Position

The standing position is clearly important for the activities of daily living. The aim of the following exercises is to add limb and thoracic movements to the stable lumbar spine and to add whole spinal movements to the stable hip. You can monitor changes in the depth of lordosis by having your client lean against a wall—feet 4-6 inches (10-15 cm) forward of the wall, his buttocks and scapulae on the wall—while you place the bladder of a pressure biofeedback unit between his lumbar spine and the wall.

Standing Sternal Lift

GOAL *To help correct excessive thoracic kyphosis by extending the thoracic spine in isolation.*

The idea of this first sequence of exercises is to teach your client to move the thoracic spine independently from the nonmoving, stable lumbar spine. Instruct your client to stand facing a table, his thighs pressed against the edge to prevent anterior shift of the pelvis into a swayback position. Have him lift the sternum up and forward, while drawing the scapulae down. Suggest that he place one hand in front of his sternum to monitor the sternal lift action. The anterior upward movement and posterior downward movement work like two guide wires pulling a wheel with its axle in the chest. The action is to flatten the thoracic curve rather than simply expand the chest or extend the lumbar spine. If your client finds it difficult to isolate the thoracic from the lumbar movement, have him try the same action while sitting—he should place his feet on a low stool to bring his knees above the level of the hips, thereby flexing the lumbar spine and reversing the lumbar lordosis. This action reduces the available extension in the lumbar spine and focuses the action to the thoracic area. After he has mastered the action in a sitting position, have him work on it while standing (see "Sternal Lift Exercise," page 162).

Pelvic Shift With Unloading

GOAL *To build isolation of leg movements on a stable base—a precursor to standing leg lifting in the frontal plane.*

Initially your client should stand with his side to a wall for support (gripping wall bars is also OK). As he develops skill in the movement, he should do it in a freestanding position. Instruct him to "lengthen his spine" ("grow taller"); to shift his pelvis to the left while maintaining alignment (a); then to unload the right leg by slightly flexing the knee and lifting the heel, while keeping the toe on the floor (b).

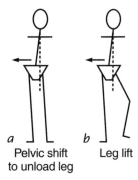

a Pelvic shift to unload leg

b Leg lift

Pelvic Shift With Leg Lift

GOAL *To teach pelvic control and stability in single-leg standing.*

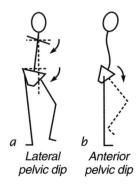

Lateral pelvic dip   *Anterior pelvic dip*

Ask your client to shift her pelvis to the left, so that her body weight is over the left leg only, then slowly lift her right leg no more than 4-6 inches (10-15 cm) while maintaining alignment *in all three planes*—there should be no posterior tilt of the pelvis, no hip drop, and no spinal rotation. Figure (a) in "Pelvic Shift With Unloading" shows the correct form; here, figure (a) shows lateral pelvic tilt (incorrect!); figure (b) illustrates anterior pelvic tilt (incorrect!). The action is one of pure hip flexion upon a stable back: the supporting leg supports the pelvis, and the pelvis supports the back. The knee should be raised no more than 45° from the horizontal. If your client finds the movement difficult to control, let her practice at first with her back supported by a wall. The sequence of pelvic shift, leg unloading, and knee lift are the same, but the back remains against the wall throughout the movement.

Standing Hip Abduction

GOAL *Learning to maintain stability in the frontal plane while performing hip abduction.*

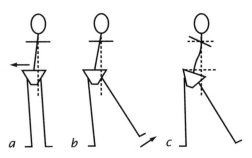

Your client begins by standing with her back 2-4 inches (5-10 cm) from a wall. If your client loses pure abduction as the movement progresses (i.e., if she uses any flexion or extension), she will know immediately because the leg will move closer to or farther away from the wall. Instruct her to shift her pelvis to the right, unloading the left leg (a). Then, maintaining alignment, she should abduct the left leg by 10-20° (b). Be sure that she does not laterally tilt her pelvis or spine (c). She should gradually increase the abduction range to a maximum of 45°. Reduce the range or stop the exercise as soon as alignment is lost.

Standing Hip Hinge

GOAL *Learning to move the spine and pelvis as a single unit on the hip.*

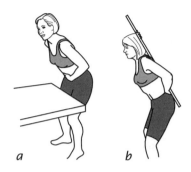

Have your client stand about 4 inches (10 cm) from a table. She may place her hands on the table only to help guide her movement, not to bear weight. Instruct her to bend from the hip, keeping her spine straight, until the spine is angled 30-45° from the vertical. It is often easier if your client focuses attention on her sacrum and imagines it moving from near vertical to near horizontal—tell her to "push her tail away." Once she has mastered this movement, she should do it without table support. Two kinds of feedback may be helpful. First, she can monitor pelvic tilt by placing the flat of one hand over the lower (infraumbilical) abdomen and the back of the other hand over the sacrum (a). The action is to tilt the pelvis while maintaining the relationship of the lumbar spine to the pelvis—the palm of the back hand should end up facing toward the ceiling. The second feedback method uses a long, straight stick. As your client places one hand over her sacrum and the other between her shoulder blades, she should grip the stick with both hands. She must keep her spine on the stick as she performs the hip hinge action (b). Rounding the spine (a typical error) increases pressure of the spinous processes on the stick; hollowing the spine increases the gap between the spine and the stick.

Exercises in the Sitting Position

Incorrect sitting positions often cause low back pain, especially that of postural origin. But, while sitting at home or work, one can also conveniently practice the following exercises throughout the day. The first exercise uses the process of relative flexibility to overload the stabilizing system.

The sitting position used in these exercises must reflect the optimal alignment of body segments. The hips should be at 70° flexion; the knees should be below the hips and slightly wider than shoulder-width apart (bringing the knees together posteriorly tilts the pelvis through soft tissue tension). About 70% of the body's weight should rest on the ischial tuberosities, 30% on the pubis. The gravity line for the upper body should pass from the center of the hip joint to the shoulder joint and ear canal, with the spine evenly distributed along the gravity line. Your instructions to hollow the abdomen and "lengthen the spine" will help bring about the correct alignment. If you wish, you can monitor the depth of the lumbar lordosis with pressure biofeedback, placing the bladder of the unit between the lumbar spine and the chair back. (Note that the sitting position used in this case is not what most people use in everyday activities; they can have their backs against the chair for use with a pressure bladder by slightly straddling the seat with their legs, which, as you recall, are to be somewhat spread, with knees lower than hips.)

Sitting Hamstring Stretch

GOAL *Maintaining pelvic position against the pull of the hamstrings.*

For the first exercise, instruct your client to straighten one leg to stretch the hamstrings, while maintaining lumbar-pelvic alignment. As soon as the pelvis posteriorly tilts (to bring the ischial tuberosity forward and take the stretch off the hamstrings), stop the exercise because alignment has been lost. Progress the exercise by gradually straightening the leg further (while maintaining alignment) until the knee can be locked fully with the hip at 70° flexion (see "Tripod Stretch," page 117).

Sitting Sternal Lift

GOAL *Performing active thoracic extension and isolating it from lumbar extension.*

Instruct your client to raise her sternum while drawing the scapulae down, as in the standing sternal lift on page 179. The movement is one of thoracic spine extension rather than deep inspiration. To assist the learning process, place the flat of your hand on your client's sternum and "draw it up," while placing the thumb and forefingers of your opposite hand on the inferior angles of the scapulae and "draw it down." If breathing control proves to be problematic, encourage your client to breathe out as she begins the sternal lift. Many people mistakenly extend the lumbar spine rather than the thoracic spine. If this occurs with your client, let her practice the exercise with her feet on a small stool to bring her knees *above* hip level—this position reverses the lumbar lordosis and throws the extension force high up the spine to the thoracic

continued

Sitting Sternal Lift, continued

region. Once she has mastered the movement in this position, try the standard position again (see "Sternal Lift Exercise," [a], page 162).

Sitting Knee Raise

GOAL *Maintaining pelvic position against the pull of the hip flexors.*

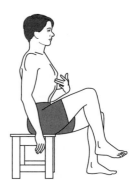

In this third exercise, we overload the stability muscles by using the pull of the iliopsoas to displace the lumbar spine. Instruct your client to raise one knee, in stages, to about 3 inches above the horizontal, while maintaining lumbar-pelvic alignment. Be sure that he avoids posterior pelvic tilt. Initially, he should gradually unload the limb by lifting just the heel. If he is able to maintain good alignment, have him proceed to lift the entire leg.

Sitting Knee and Arm Raise

GOAL *Increasing the complexity to challenge coordination.*

Have your client flex one arm to 90°. Holding a small (7.5-10 lb., or 3-5 kg) dumbbell in the hand increases the overload; he should keep the dumbbell moving rather than holding it still. Combining alternate arm and leg movements is a useful progression—the right arm is lifted at the same time as the left knee to provide a diagonal stress on the body; this is then reversed with the left arm and right knee being raised.

Repeated Pelvic Tilting Exercises Using Balance Boards

Moving the pelvis beneath an immobile trunk is an excellent teaching method to improve control of the neutral position, to reduce muscle reaction speed, and to enhance general stability. Using a "rocker board" (moves like a see-saw), and progressing to a "wobble board" (mounted on a hemisphere—moves in any direction), is an effective (and rather fun) way to perform such exercises.

Simple Pelvic Tilt, Progressing to Use of Balance Boards

GOAL *For advanced control of pelvic tilt.*

At first, have your client sit in the optimal position (see page 181) on a wooden bench or stool with his feet on the floor. Instruct him to tilt his pelvis alternately in the anterior and then posterior direction, while maintaining the position of his shoulders and thoracic spine. The aim is to isolate the pelvis and lower lumbar spine from the thoracic spine, and the shoulders from the upper lumbar spine. Progress the exercise by having your client perform it while sitting first on a rocker board (like a see-saw, moves in only one plane—shown in the next exercise section), and then on a wobble board (mounted on a sphere, moves in any direction—see page 185, "Neutral Position Maintenance").

Pelvic Rock on Rocker Board

GOAL *Progression from simple pelvic tilt.*

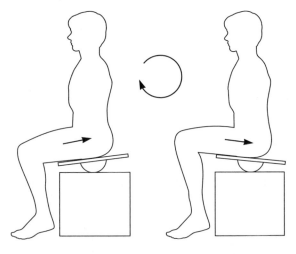

Initially place the rocker in the frontal plane to facilitate anterior and posterior tilting of the pelvis. Changing the rocker orientation of the board to the sagittal plane will facilitate lateral tilting. In each case, the lumbar-pelvic movement must be isolated from that of the upper body. To begin working for muscle reaction speed, apply pressure on the shoulders to push your client off balance while he tries to stay upright on the rocker board. Alternate the orientation of the board, between frontal and sagittal planes. You'll know when to stop any given session when your client is no longer able to maintain neutral position or maintain abdominal hollowing. Build up to 2 minutes in both planes before progressing to the wobble board.

Pelvic Rock on Wobble Board

GOAL *Multiplane (sagittal, frontal, and transverse) stability in sitting.*

Initially, have your client merely sit on the wobble board and attempt to maintain the optimal sitting position. Have him progress to single plane actions (flexion/extension and lateral flexion). Once he has mastered these actions, instruct him to "tip the board around a clock face" (i.e., to tilt to 1 o'clock and then back to neutral, to 2 o'clock and back to neutral, to 3 o'clock and back to neutral, etc.). Encourage him to use slow, deliberate movements, taking perhaps 2-5 seconds to reach each position of the clock, holding that position for 2 seconds, taking 2-5 seconds to return to neutral, holding neutral position for 2 seconds, and then beginning the next phase.

Neutral Position Maintenance

GOAL *Building stability reaction speed in sitting.*

Finally, you should try to knock your client off balance while he maintains the neutral position on a wobble board. Initially use slow-onset pressure, working gradually up to rapid pressure from a variety of directions. Have your client close his eyes to facilitate anticipatory muscle action and muscle contraction speed. The progression here is one of time. Initially, try to prolong the movement for 30 seconds, then 60 seconds, stopping each time when alignment is lost or the client loses his balance.

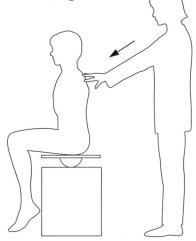

Sitting Hip Hinge

GOAL *Moving spine and pelvis as a single unit on the hip.*

The final exercise is the hip hinge (compare "Standing Hip Hinge," page 181). As in all these sitting exercises, be sure your client begins

continued

Sitting Hip Hinge, continued

in the optimal sitting position, with the knees astride to facilitate pelvic tilt (see description under "Exercises in the Sitting Position," page 181). Have him tip the whole of his upper body forward as a single unit, moving the pelvis and spine on the fixed femur. He should initiate the action by leaning his whole body forward to change the sitting weight distribution. In optimal sitting, approximately 30% of the body weight is taken on the pubic bones and 70% on the ischial tuberosities, provided that the knees are aligned below the hip and the femurs are angled below the horizontal. As your client leans forward, he takes weight from the ischial tuberosities and places it onto the pubic bone, ending with 70-80% of his weight on the pubic bone. To lean back, he reverses the weight transference. To facilitate the action, suggest that he perform it while sitting on a rocker board. In each case the pelvis and spine should move as one unit, avoiding any change in lordosis.

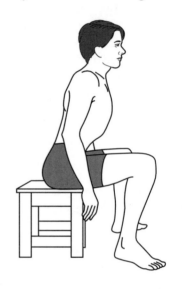

STABILITY BALL EXERCISES

In addition to or even instead of the exercises in the previous section, your clients can obtain advanced levels of stability by exercises with stability balls (also called gym balls). These exercises require quite complex movements and will help increase the stability already obtained through previous exercises in this book. They also can strengthen stability muscles that otherwise might not be exercised.

At first your clients should use the ball under your supervision, but later they can use it at home—it is an inexpensive and effective apparatus for back stability. Several authors have described general exercises on the gym ball, and these publications make useful follow-up material (Hyman and Liebenson 1996; Lester and Posner-Mayer 1993; Norris 1995a).

A 26-inch (65-cm) gym ball facilitates the optimal sitting position for most people. Your clients should be able to sit on the ball with their femurs horizontal and their hips and knees both at approximately 90° flexion. Feet should be shoulder-width apart and flat on the floor to enable free pelvic tilting and provide a wide base of support. The ball should be inflated so that it feels firm but will give slightly when a person sits on it. Use higher inflation pressures for heavier clients. Deflating the ball slightly will increase the base of support.

You can reduce the ball's tendency to roll by setting it on a "collar"—a plastic ring on the floor. When you need to increase your clients' confidence or provide support, place the ball between two chairs: either position the chair backs toward the ball so that your clients can lightly touch the chair with arms outstretched at shoulder level; or, for even more support, position the seats toward the ball so your clients can place the flats of their hands on the seat surface.

As with all exercises, your clients should warm up and stretch before engaging in these activities. During all exercises they should maintain the neutral position of their spines and keep their abdomens hollowed. They should perform mirror images of any one-sided exercises, so the body is worked symmetrically.

The progression with stability ball exercises is similar to that for previous exercises: begin with 8-10 repetitions, for example, then increase to 12-15. Note that the gym ball introduces balance as an additional variable. Even if your clients are not fatigued, if they lose alignment or lose their balance and become unstable (and therefore likely to slip off the ball), they must stop, rest, and start again using a lower number of repetitions. If gym ball exercises are the only ones your clients are doing, they should perform all of the following exercises during each session. I suggest at least three but no more than five sessions per week, for at least 10-16 weeks. At first have your clients use a slow count of 4 or 5 to move into the holding position; hold the designated position for a count of 5; then use a count of 4 or 5 to move back into the starting position. They can progress by adding reps and/or by adding to the holding time. Determine the limits for a given exercise by observing the point at which your clients just begin to lose spinal alignment or abdominal hollowing, or to lose their balance—then instruct them to stay just below that level of timing or rep number for at least a week before trying to add holding time or reps. They should always stay just a little bit within their maximum capacity, as determined by their ability to maintain alignment and abdominal hollowing.

Sitting Knee Raise

GOAL *Maintaining stability in the presence of hip movement on a reduced base of support.*

While sitting upright on the gym ball, your client should lift a single knee from 90° hip flexion to 120° hip flexion. She must make the action slow and deliberate, maintaining her body position throughout, and avoiding the temptation to "fall toward" the lifting leg.

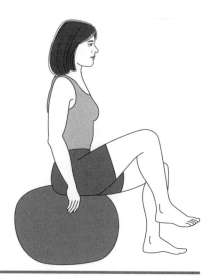

Abdominal Slide

GOAL *Controlling the action of the rectus abdominis while moving.*

Instruct your client to tilt her pelvis backward from a sitting position on the ball, then to roll back until her spine rests on the ball. The action is to roll through the spine—the ischial tuberosities begin on the ball, but the weight is transferred to the coccyx and sacrum and eventually to the lumbar spine. The final holding position is with the trunk slightly flexed and the abdominal muscles contracted in a half-sitting position.

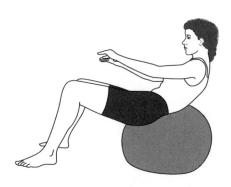

Half-Sitting Arm and Leg Movements

GOAL *Maintaining stability while moving arms and legs in an unstable position.*

continued

Half-Sitting Arm and Leg Movements, continued

Have your client perform the abdominal slide action just described, but maintain the position when his trunk is at 45° to the horizontal. Then he should raise one arm while lowering the other. Once he can do this in a controlled fashion, with the trunk remaining in alignment, have him rest his arms, then lift one leg while lowering the other. He should try to keep the thigh of the leg being raised parallel to the ground (i.e., only the lower leg should move). Finally, he should perform arm and leg movements together—the right arm and left leg lifting together, and vice versa. To make the exercise even more challenging, suggest that your client hold small dumbbells in his hands as he does the movements.

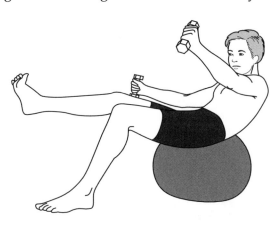

Lying Trunk Curl Over Ball

GOAL *Strengthens upper rectus abdominis muscles.*

Instruct your client to begin with his thoracolumbar spine supported on the ball, his arms at his side. He should move from this slightly flexed position to spinal extension, relaxing over the ball. He then performs a curling movement while performing abdominal hollowing and pressing his lumbar spine onto the ball surface. Once he can perform the basic exercise well, increase the difficulty by having him hold his arms by the side of his head or even completely overhead.

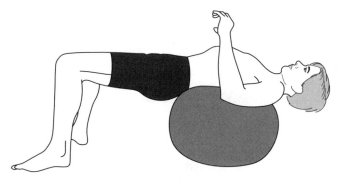

Lying Trunk Curl With Leg Lift

GOAL *Strengthens upper and lower abdominals.*

From the "lying trunk curl over ball" position, your client should lift one leg while maintaining the stable position, trying to keep the thigh parallel to the other thigh. The 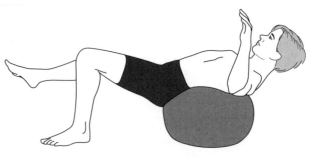 movement is easier if the ball rests closer to the shoulders with the waist at the ball's edge rather than at the ball's center. Lying over the ball, in fact, is an excellent way to *stretch* the whole spine into extension as part of postural correction of a flatback posture.

Basic Superman

GOAL *Strengthens the spinal and hip extensors.*

Have your client lie prone with his abdomen on the ball, and his feet astride and flat against a wall. He should tighten his abdominal muscles to form a firm surface pressing against the ball and retract his head (tuck the chin in without looking down). He should retract and depress his shoulders in order to draw his arms downward and back, then extend his thoracic spine to bring his chest off the ball. Have him hold the inner-range position for 5-10 seconds.

Superman With Arms

GOAL *Strengthens spinal extensors; helps shoulder retractors contribute more to movement.*

From the basic superman movement, instruct your client to extend first one and then both arms overhead to increase the overload for both trunk and shoulders. Holding a light ball or balloon between his hands can help give him the feeling of lengthening his body. Observe carefully to make sure that your client doesn't lose alignment and hyperextend his spine. There should be a straight line through the heels, knees, hips, shoulders, and hands.

continued

Superman With Arms, continued

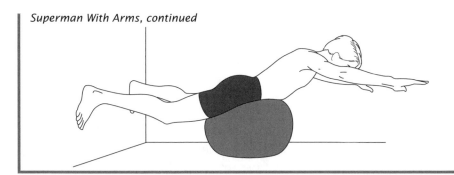

Bridge

GOAL *To simultaneously strengthen both hip extensors and spinal extensors.*

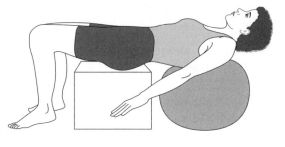

Have your client lie with her shoulders and back on the ball and her feet flat on the floor, knees apart. At first, place a small stool under her buttocks and instruct her to raise and lower her body from the stool using hip extension force. Once she is able to hold the raised position, remove the stool. Instruct her to hold the position, making sure that her lumbar spine is in its optimal position; she should gradually build up the holding time to 30 seconds.

Bridge With Pelvic Tilt

GOAL *Strengthens back and hip extensors while improving control of pelvic tilt.*

While your client holds the bridge position, have her perform a *pelvic tilt*. She can intensify the bridge movement by combining anterior tilt with lowering her buttocks onto the floor, and a posterior tilt with lifting herself back into the bridge position. This exercise helps teach the subtleties of muscle control involved in minor adjustments in pelvic tilt. It is especially helpful to clients who can only perform a tilt as an "all-or-nothing" movement using maximal force to bring about a full tilt.

Bridge With Leg Lift

GOAL *Increases overload—especially of lower abdominals—during bridge.*

Have your client perform the standard bridge exercise—but once he is in the high position, he should lift one knee to bring the foot off the ground. Be sure that he maintains spinal alignment, avoiding the temptation to tip the pelvis toward the lifted leg. If he finds it difficult to keep his pelvis level, place a stick across the front of the pelvis just below the level of the anterior superior iliac spines. If the pelvis tilts too far, the stick will fall off!

Bridge With Leg Lift and Extension

GOAL *Strengthens lower abdominals while increasing leg control.*

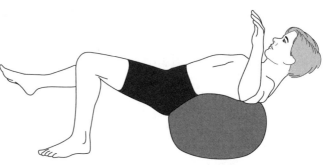

Have your client perform the standard bridge and lift the right knee so that the right foot clears the floor, avoiding the tendency to allow the pelvis to tilt to the right.

At the high position, he should gradually straighten the right leg until it is completely in line with the spine. After maintaining this position for 2-3 seconds, he slowly bends the leg and lowers it till his foot is back on the ground.

Bridge With Therapist Pressure

GOAL *Strengthens hip and trunk stability muscles by challenging stability with continuously variable overload from multiple directions.*

While your client performs the standard bridge, you should kneel at his side. Push against his pelvis from above/below and side/side. Rapid pushes will decrease muscle reaction time, training the muscles to contract more quickly without loss of intensity.

Reverse Bridge

GOAL *Strengthens back and hip muscles while increasing leg motion control.*

Your client's feet and calves should rest on the ball, with her trunk on the floor. Instruct her to abduct her arms to about 30° to aid balance. Then she should lift her hips to make a straight line from the shoulders to the hips and feet.

Reverse Bridge and Roll

GOAL *Strengthens trunk and hip muscles, while increasing leg motion control.*

Once your client is in the high position of the reverse bridge movement, she should roll the ball toward herself by flexing her knees and hips; then roll it away by extending the legs again.

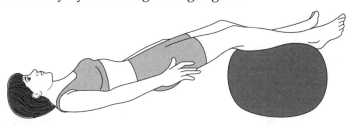

Heel Bridge

GOAL *Increases overload in the bridge position.*

Instruct your client to assume the high position of the reverse bridge, with this difference: only her 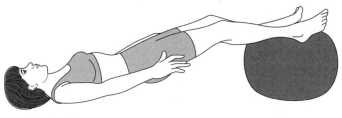 heels should be on the ball. Instruct her to push each heel alternately into the ball—this entails pushing down with the whole leg to activate the hamstrings and gluteals, rather than simply flexing the knee to work the hamstrings alone.

Single-Leg Heel Bridge

GOAL *Provides maximal overload in the bridge position.*

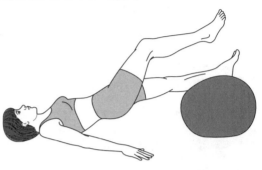

Your client's trunk should be on the floor, and only her heels should be on the ball. Have her lift one leg and hold it away from the ball. Then have her perform a single-leg heel bridge by pushing her heel into the ball and lifting her buttocks off the floor. She should hold the position for 5-10 seconds, then lower her body under control to the starting position.

Heel Bridge With Leg Raise, Ball Rolling

GOAL *Provides maximal overload in the bridge position, while increasing leg movement control.*

Instruct your client to begin as with the previous exercise, up through the point of raising one leg. At this point, she should roll the ball toward herself by flexing her knee and hip; then roll it away by extending her leg again.

Prone Fall

GOAL *Provides co-contraction for the hip and trunk muscles.*

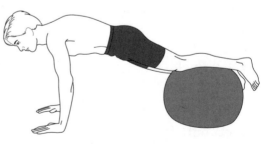

Have your client place his thighs on the ball, with his legs together and his hands on the floor. He should lengthen his body to achieve a neutral spine, and retract his head to maintain cervical alignment. He should begin with the ball close to his pelvis, and then walk his hands forward so that the ball moves down his legs toward the knees. By shifting the body's center of gravity farther from the center of the ball, this movement increases the leverage effect.

Prone Fall With Arm Lift

GOAL *Increases overload in prone fall.*

Have your client begin with the prone fall movement. Then he should lift one hand about 0.5 inches (1.3 cm) from the floor without allowing the shoulder girdle to dip down. He then lifts the arm first to the side and eventually forward, pointing the hand and lengthening the whole body.

Prone Fall With Single-Leg Lift

GOAL *Increases overload (especially for gluteals) in prone fall, while training for abdominal-gluteal co-contraction.*

Have your client begin with the prone fall movement, then lift one leg to 15° hip extension, keeping the knee locked. Instruct him to perform alternate single-leg lifts; to train for speed as well as strength, have him gradually increase the speed of the lifts. Eventually he should do them as fast as he can without losing correct alignment.

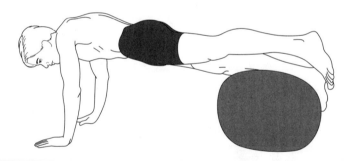

Wall Sit

GOAL *To prepare the body for lifting, while strengthening the legs to provide power for the lift.*

Your client performs the following exercise with the ball sandwiched between his back and a wall. This has two main advantages over simply leaning against the wall. First, vertical movement is easier because the rolling of the ball removes the friction between the individual's back

continued

Wall Sit, continued

and the wall. Second, these exercises require more control since the subject is leaning on a mobile object rather than a fixed wall. The greater degree of control builds more automatic stability (i.e., the individual need not focus so much on the stability muscles in order to keep them stable).

While your client stands with his back toward the wall, his feet about 2.5 feet (0.75 m) from the wall, place the gym ball between the wall and the lumbar region of his back. Instruct him to lower his body to the sitting position while rolling the ball down the wall. Once he achieves 90° hip and knee flexion (a), he should hold the position for 5-10 seconds and then roll back up to the starting position. He can then progress to the single-leg wall sit (b).

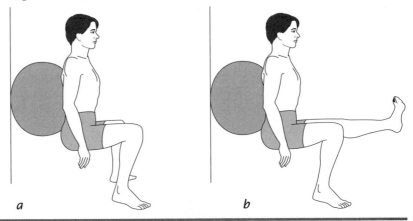

a   b

Free Squat

GOAL *Teaches whole-body control during vertical movement.*

Place the gym ball on a collar to stop it from rolling. Have your client stand in front of the ball, feet astride. She should slowly squat, keeping her back aligned, until she sits on the ball, then slowly stand up again.

Arm Lift in 4-Point Kneeling

GOAL *Increases overall stability during shoulder movements.*

Decrease the ball pressure for kneeling actions so that it will fit comfortably under your client's abdomen in 4-point kneeling. Once your client is kneeling over the ball, instruct him to lift first one (a) and then both

continued

Arm Lift in 4-Point Kneeling, continued

arms to the horizontal. Tell him to "lengthen his body" through the arms and hold the fully extended position for 5-10 seconds. The next progression is for the client to extend his spine and lift his arms behind himself to the horizontal (b).

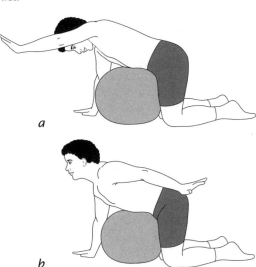

a

b

Double-Leg Raise

GOAL *Increases strength of hip and spine extensors, while promoting trunk stability.*

Your client begins as with the previous exercise, but with the ball lower down the body toward the hips. Have him first lift one leg to the horizontal, maintaining good body alignment throughout the action.

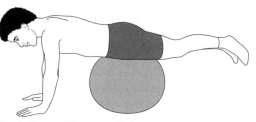

He can then progress to lifting both legs. If your client's legs are especially heavy, his arms may lift from the floor during this exercise. To prevent this, he should hold onto a low object such as the legs of a heavy gym bench. He should hold the fully extended position for 5-10 seconds.

PROPRIOCEPTIVE TRAINING

The aim of most of the training in this book is for your clients (1) to learn to move/position their muscles in such a way that their lower backs will become stable, and (2) to *keep* their backs in the stable position. And the second goal is virtually unattainable unless your clients' bodies learn to do what is necessary without conscious thought. The movements, the postures, and the balance must be more automatic. This is the goal of proprioceptive training.

Theory of Proprioception

Because I believe it is important that you know the underlying mechanisms behind the activities you prescribe for your clients, the next few paragraphs provide a brief overview of proprioception.

Movement Sense

Kinesthetic awareness, or "movement sense," includes the detection of both joint displacement and change in velocity (i.e., acceleration). It is commonly assessed by measuring *the threshold to detection of passive motion* (TTDPM): individuals simply state when they feel movement has begun. One cannot act to correct imbalance until one is aware that there is an imbalance. The awareness can be conscious or unconscious, however, and the corrective action likewise can be intentional or automatic. The purpose of proprioceptive training is to help individuals learn both to detect and to correct imbalances without conscious awareness that they are doing so. Consciously performed joint-positioning activities, especially at end range, will enhance the development of automatic control and cognitive awareness (Lephart and Fu 1995).

Regulation of Muscle Stiffness

Dynamic joint stability (i.e., the body's ability to constantly make unconscious "microcorrections" to keep a joint stable) occurs via reflexes at the spinal level. And reflexes by definition are not conscious or intentional movements. A common illustration is the body's response when your finger touches a hot skillet. The incoming nerve stimulus (*afferent*, i.e., going "toward" the central nervous system) doesn't even make it to the brain—rather, it gets only as far as the spinal cord before it is processed and an appropriate outgoing (*efferent*, i.e., going "away from" the central nervous system) signal is sent to the muscles: "Move your hand!" In fact, you end up moving your hand *without thinking about it* because your brain had nothing to do with the reaction—it all occurred in a "closed loop" of signals between your hand and your spinal cord.

The ideal situation as far as back stability is concerned is that you have such "closed loop" efferent signals constantly going out to your stability muscles: the receptor nerves detect a slight increase in instability, they send messages to the spinal cord, and instantaneously outgoing "efferent" signals are sent out to tweak a multifidus muscle, to slightly increase tension in your left internal oblique muscle, etc. It all happens dozens of times a second without your even thinking about it.

Such is the goal of proprioceptive exercises. It is possible to "train" your nervous system to be more sensitive to incoming messages that say "stability is weakening" and to provide more *automatic* outgoing signals that instruct which muscles to change in which way. If such a fine-tuned system seems unimaginable, try this experiment: open a water faucet at least halfway, place a drinking glass under it, and keep the glass as perfectly level as you can. You'll find that you can keep it quite still. Now consider the complexity of the nerve signals involved in the task you just completed. Thousands of times a second, afferent signals left your hand with the message, "The cup has just gotten heavier." And thousands of times a second, efferent signals returned from your central nervous system: "OK, tighten such-and-such muscles a teensy bit more." But it all happens so fast, and the microadjustments are so smooth, that for the most part your hand is able to hold the drinking glass *stable*. This is a closed loop system. Your brain isn't significantly involved. The signals go to your spinal cord, they are processed, and the return messages head immediately back to your hand.

Proprioceptive exercises involve sudden alterations in joint position in order to train the body's reflexes. Chapter 7 provided exercises to help your clients learn simply to reproduce passive positioning of body segments. The training in this section is similar to those activities, but on a *very* fast track! In order to thoroughly follow an individual's progress, you theoretically can measure the precise onset of muscle contraction in relation to joint displacement—unfortunately, however, you most likely would need to refer your client to a physical therapy department or specialist biomechanics lab to make accurate measurements. Yet, with experience, you can assess onset of muscle contraction to some degree by palpating the muscle during a passive movement test. This type of examination, while not exact, can be useful for muscle re-education. The aim is simply to note if the muscles are able to limit joint displacement and effectively stabilize the joint.

Benefits of Training

Using TTDPM and reproduction of passive positioning (RPP), Barrack et al. (1983) found decreased kinesthesia with increasing age (i.e., the closed loop system for stability works less well). Injury further reduces proprioceptive input due to prolonged inactivity and damage to proprioceptive nerve endings within the injured tissues. A number of authors have stressed the importance of proprioceptive training in rehabilitation following injury to the knee (Barrack et al. 1983; Beard et al. 1994), ankle (Freeman et al. 1965; Konradsen and Ravn 1990; Lentell et al. 1990), and shoulder

(Lephart et al. 1994; Smith and Brunolli 1990). The functional importance of proprioceptive training has also been emphasized during rehabilitation of the spine (Irion 1992; Lewit 1991; Norris 1995a), although its use in spinal rehabilitation is less common than for other areas of the body.

Proprioception and accompanying reflexes may indeed be enhanced with training. Barrack et al. (1983) found enhanced kinesthesia in trained dancers, and Lephart and Fu (1995) demonstrated the same in intercollegiate gymnasts. Both types of athletes practice free exercise using body weight as resistance and using complex multijoint activities. This type of training appears appropriate for proprioceptive rehabilitation.

> **KEY POINT:** Proprioception and stabilizing reflexes may be enhanced by using training that involves complex multijoint activities.

The basis of proprioceptive training for the back is maintenance of stability *against a rapidly applied force tending to displace the spine*. In most cases, you can instruct your clients to practice one or more of the following exercises for at least five minutes a day, four or five days per week. The limiting factor is whether or not your clients can keep their spines stable (they should stop before they lose stability). They should do the most advanced exercise(s) of which they are capable, as quickly as they are able—remember, the idea is to train their reflexes to act with such extreme speed that maintaining spinal stability will be as smooth an operation as your holding the glass motionless as it fills under a tap.

Rapid Displacement in Sitting

GOAL *Develop muscle reaction speed for back stability.*

Have your client sit on a stool with her spine optimally aligned. A training partner stands behind her and presses against her shoulders from multiple directions to flex, extend, and laterally flex the spine. Initially the pressure should be even, but gradually it should become varied in both direction and force. The aim is for your client to be able to rapidly stabilize the spine *before* the spine moves away from its neutral position. Instruct her to relax her trunk muscles between repetitions (which should last about a minute each), rather than hold them rigidly braced throughout the whole exercise. If you have it available, you may want to use surface EMG to monitor changing muscle tone. As your client's reactions become more proficient, the movements should become faster—but she must always maintain good alignment.

Muscle Reaction Speed Using a Mobile Platform

GOAL *Further develop muscle reaction speed for back stability.*

Instruct your client to assume a 2-point kneeling position on a balance board and to align his lumbar spine into its neutral position. Then a training partner should push him off balance so that the platform tilts. The aim is to maintain lumbar stability as the board tilts, *while keeping the edges of the board off the ground.* Start with a rocker board (allows single-plane motion), advancing later to a domed balance board (wobble board) that allows triplane motion. You may also want to use other mobile platforms such as the Fitter ski trainer (Fitter International Inc., Calgary, Alberta, Canada), the slide trainer (Forza Fitness Equipment, London, England), or a mini trampette (available in most large sports stores). Again, increase the speed of the movements as your client becomes more proficient.

Throw-Catch Activities on a Mobile Surface

GOAL *Develop rapid-onset back stability.*

Throw-catch activities using a basketball or medicine ball will increase the challenge to the stabilizing system. The aim is to align the lumbar spine optimally while balancing on the mobile surface. As your client catches the ball, she must maintain spinal alignment in spite of the platform's motion. Instruct your client to increase the speed of the exercises as she becomes more proficient.

SUMMARY

- Once individuals have achieved basic back stability through the exercises in previous chapters, they can begin building greater stability and training their backs for sports or on-the-job lifting by using the advanced exercises in this chapter.
- Advanced stability exercises, with movement of limbs on the stable trunk, will greatly increase an individual's ability to maintain back stability *automatically*, without conscious thought.
- Exercises with gym balls also help develop automatic stability and help develop muscles that previous, more basic, exercises may not affect.
- Proprioceptive exercises can be very useful in training your clients' reflexes to automatically (unconsciously) keep the spine stable.

9

More Advanced
Stability Training:
Weight Training and Plyometrics

If one's goal is merely to develop adequate back stability, special equipment is unnecessary. People with sport and occupational injuries, however, require *limb strength* in addition to back stability in order to complete their rehabilitation—especially if they are to resume on-the-job lifting tasks or sports activities in which the body works against resistance.

Weight training has several important advantages for those with lower back problems. First, it can increase the limb strength that some people need. Second, it can further enhance trunk muscle strength/stability to the level often required in sports—especially contact sports where abdominal strength can have a protective function for the internal organs. Finally, weight training can help to guard against further back injury.

When we use weight training for back stability, we are strengthening muscles upon an already stable base—weight training is appropriate *only* for individuals who have already re-educated and built up endurance within the stabilizing muscles. Weight training takes the process further, adding greater resistance both to strengthen muscle and to challenge the stability system itself. The target muscles are those of the trunk, the limb muscles attaching to the trunk, and the limb muscles that provide the power for lifting.

Plyometric exercises also can enhance strength and stability, with the added benefit of training for very fast reaction times. Your clients can use plyometrics in place of weight training if they wish, although I suggest a combination of both if they can afford the time. They need good stability before beginning either kind of training—but since the speed of movement in plyometrics is far greater than that in basic weight training, your clients will need better stability to begin plyometrics than to begin using machine weights.

> **KEY POINT:** Weight training or plyometric exercise for greater back stability is appropriate *only* for those who have already developed good back stability using exercises described earlier in this book.

WEIGHT TRAINING

Emphasize to your clients that the weight training you are giving them is specifically part of a back stability program, and therefore the activities will be somewhat different from those they may see other people doing in the weight rooms. Make sure they understand that they must follow *your* instructions, resisting the temptation to emulate the practices of other exercisers.

Before You Start

Before introducing any of these weight-training exercises, give your clients the following instructions: (1) They must keep the whole spine correctly aligned and the lumbar spine in neutral position. (2) They should perform abdominal hollowing to tighten the stabilizing muscles and provide a stable base upon which the limbs can move. (3) They should exhale when lifting a weight, rather than holding their breaths, and be careful that deep breathing does not lead to hyperventilation and associated dizziness.

Weight training involves three types of muscle work. The weight is lifted through *concentric* muscle action, held steady by *isometric* action, and lowered under control by *eccentric* action. Your clients should use all three phases. Remind them that the common practice of lifting the weight rapidly and then dropping it minimizes eccentric and isometric action, both of which are vital to stability work. A ratio of lifting for a count of 3, holding for a count of 2, and lowering for a count of 4 will emphasize each type of muscle work.

Your clients should feel comfortably challenged during these exercises rather than excessively strained. Their breathing rates will increase, but they should be able to talk normally at all times—if they are fighting for breath, the exercise intensity is too great for rehabilitation and you should stop the exercise. Individuals may sweat lightly and experience mild reddening/darkening of the skin; but excessive red coloration and bulging of veins in the face and neck are indications that the exercise intensity is too great, and the exercise should be stopped. See that a therapist or trainer supervises your clients during the initial stages of weight training, until both parties are confident that the exercise techniques are correct.

Safety Check

All exercise equipment has risks that must be minimized (see "Safety Checklist for Weight Training," below). The risks fall broadly into two categories: those associated with moving machinery, and those associated with the lifting action itself. Here are the rules you should present to your clients, and the explanations you should give them for why the rules are important:

• **Control the weights.** Moving weights carry considerable momentum. Unless the weights are kept under control throughout the full range of motion, there is considerable risk to joints and body tissues. When a limb reaches the end of its motion range, the ligaments and muscles surrounding it become tight and limit further movement. Movements that are too rapid lead to loss of control—the joint stops moving at the end of the motion range, but the inertia of the weight forces the joint further against the tightening support tissues, causing severe trauma or overuse injury. With a **traumatic injury,** tissues are suddenly torn and function is lost—the athlete sometimes feels the body part "tear" or "give." Bleeding and swelling result. **Overuse injuries** are more insidious. The tissues undergo microtrauma as they are continually pulled further than their normal range allows. The resulting low-grade inflammation in some cases gives rise to formation of scar tissue, and in others may actually pull a tendon attachment away from the bone. When this happens the bone membrane (periosteum) may be lifted and the area may calcify, giving a cloudy appearance on X ray. In either case, the message is clear: when using

---

Safety Checklist for Weight Training

- Always warm up before training.
- Check machinery before use.
- Set up machinery to suit your height and weight.
- Tie back long hair and be careful with loose clothing.
- Remove jewelry.
- Wear serviceable footwear—*no flip-flops!*
- Use correct exercise techniques and keep the weight under control.
- Watch your body alignment—keep a neutral, stable spine.
- Keep abdomen hollowed during exercises.
- Practice good back care—lift correctly.
- Train within your own limitations.
- Never train through an injury—*see a physical therapist.*

Adapted, by permission, from C.M. Norris, 1995, *Weight training: Principles and practice* (London: A & C Black).

weight-training apparatus, your clients must always move the weights in a controlled fashion.

> **KEY POINT:** When using weight-training equipment, your clients must move the weights in a controlled, slow manner. Tell them, "Make sure you control the weight; don't let it control you!"

• **Wear appropriate clothing.** Even though most machines have guards, fingers and especially hair and clothing can be trapped in the moving weight stack with severe results. Instruct your clients to tie back long hair when they use machine weights and to keep loose clothing well away from the machines. They should remove watches, large rings, and dangling jewelry. Good sports shoes will help protect their feet—the weight gym is no place for beach shoes or flip-flops! Toes can be stubbed and free weights dropped onto feet. As well as giving your lower limbs better alignment, sports shoes offer the first line of defense against foot injuries.

• **Adjust the equipment.** Most good weight-training machines allow users to adjust the unit for the shape and size of their bodies. Make sure that the machine is set up *before* it is used, and that the user knows exactly how the machine works before beginning the exercise.

• **Know your limits.** Remind your clients to train *well within* their limits. An old adage says, "Never sacrifice technique for weight." Lifting a weight that is too heavy can impair both technique and body alignment and increase the risk of injury.

• **Listen to your body.** Your clients must not train with an injury unless they are following a structured rehabilitation program. The key is to listen to the body, especially pain. Never allow an individual to exercise through *increasing* pain. If a movement hurts and is continued slowly, the pain may diminish—in which case the person is probably suffering from stiffness that is working loose. If pain increases, however, the movement must stop. Caution: remember that some rapid, repeated actions may "reduce" pain simply because the exercise hurts more than the injury! Alert your clients to this possibility, and remind them to stop such movements immediately if they even suspect a masking effect.

> **KEY POINT:** Never exercise through increasing pain.

Machine Exercises

A major advantage of machine exercises is that they usually allow only single-plane motions and are therefore easy to coordinate (pulleys are an exception—

because they allow motion in three planes, they require more complex coordination). Have your clients use "pyramid training," with light resistance for the first sets to prepare the muscles for higher overload. They generally should employ slow repetitions to make the movement exact, and light resistances in order to build endurance. Obviously, they should do all exercises using both left and right sides of their bodies—they should simply follow mirror-image instructions for any one-sided exercises described in the next section.

Once your clients have mastered the basic movements for any of these exercises, using fairly light weights, prescribe a progressive program similar to the following, taking your clients' individual needs into account: for each machine, determine the weight with which the clients can perform 15 full repetitions and still have enough energy left to do 3 or 4 more before reaching exhaustion. Prescribe 12-15 reps per exercise session, three sessions per week, skipping at least one day between sessions. After two weeks, they can increase the weight, again according to how much they can lift using 15 full reps and not quite be at the point of exhaustion. Let them follow this program—12-15 reps/session, three sessions/week, for a period of at least 16 weeks, never increasing the weights past the point where they can do 15 reps and still feel they can do several more. Remember, this is not a program of building photogenic bodies—it is a program designed to further increase back stability and help prevent future back problems.

You can prescribe higher numbers of repetitions (20-25) to enhance muscle *endurance* rather than *strength*. Although 12-15 repetitions will produce some increase in both muscle strength and muscle endurance, higher numbers of reps are required for muscle endurance with minimal joint loading. This is relevant for clients whose clinical conditions preclude their handling larger weights. Those with high blood pressure or severe osteoporosis, for example, may require higher numbers of repetitions with very little resistance. This type of workout will help your clients learn the proper movement without overloading the joints.

The weight your clients lift should *always* feel comfortable and lightly challenging to them. If a weight feels too heavy, it will lead to poor exercise technique—and body alignment will suffer. If you see this happening, *reduce the weight*.

Lateral Pulldown

GOAL *To strengthen the latissimus dorsi (which tensions the thoracolumbar fascia, an essential component of stabilization).*

For the lat pulldown, one may lower the bar either behind the shoulders or to sternal level on the chest. Either position can be used, and both have

continued

Lateral Pulldown, continued

advantages and disadvantages. Pulling the bar behind the neck will increase your client's shoulder mobility, as that position requires a higher degree of external rotation at the shoulder than pulling the bar to the chest. Since external rotation is often limited, this is a desirable form of mobility training. Remember, however, that the seventh cervical vertebra has a very prominent spinous process (the point of bone pressing out through the skin), and your clients must take care not to strike this point with the bar. To lessen the likelihood of this happening, they should pass the bar behind the head by 2-3 inches (5-8 cm) 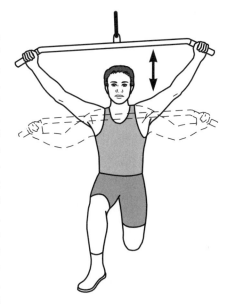 rather than letting it brush the hair. In this way, the bar will miss the cervical spine and come to rest across the shoulders. Individuals unable to adopt this position should pull the bar to the upper chest. The action is a smooth pull downward, placing the bar (in the first case) behind the neck and across the shoulders. The head should be tilted forward slightly, and the bar must not strike the cervical vertebrae but rest across the middle fibers of the trapezius. The lowering action of the weight pulls the bar up again. Instruct your clients not to permit the weights to rest together at the end of the movement, so that useful traction will be maintained in the latissimus dorsi and the thoracolumbar fascia.

Bringing the bar in front of the body to the top of the sternum reduces the range of external rotation and extension at the shoulder and is especially useful for less flexible individuals and those with a history of shoulder subluxation or dislocation. Although you may permit your clients to use whatever grip seems most comfortable—wide, narrow, pronated, supinated, or midposition—keep the following in mind: using a narrow grip either on a standard wide bar or a box frame (with elbows in pronated or midposition) will allow the elbows to pass close to the sides of the body as the bar is pulled down; and, according to Weider (1989), keeping the elbows in will thicken the latissimus dorsi rather than broaden it. Using a supinated grip reduces the emphasis on the latissimus dorsi and emphasizes the biceps brachii.

Cable Crossover

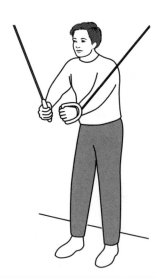

GOAL *To strengthen the latissimus dorsi and pectoralis major.*

The movement begins with both arms abducted. The feet are apart, slightly wider than shoulder width. The action is to exhale and pull both arms into adduction to the sides of the body. An alternate approach is to pull the arms forward across the chest—this technique increases the adduction range and emphasizes the pectoralis major. The elbows should be slightly bent throughout the movement, to reduce stress on the elbow joint.

Back Extension (Machine)

GOAL *Strengthens the erector spinae (full range).*

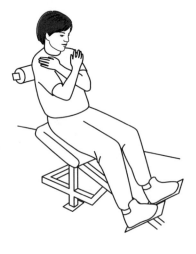

The back extension machine can help rehabilitate and strengthen the back extensors but can cause problems if faulty technique is used. It requires close supervision. Permit clients to use this machine only after they have mastered the *hip hinge action* and *pelvic tilt* movements (both in chapter 4). Have your client adjust the machine so that knees and hips are bent to 70-80° and the pivot point of the machine is aligned with the hip joint axis. The movement begins with a posterior tilt of the pelvis, moving the seat contact point from the ischial tuberosities back onto the sacrum. The action is movement of the pelvis on the stationary femur, with the back stabilized and immobile throughout the early part of the movement. Only when the second half of the movement range begins should the spine move into extension.

Back Extension (Frame)

GOAL *Strengthens the erector spinae (limited range).*

The back hyperextension frame is useful in both the early and advanced stages of training but can be dangerous if used incorrectly. The exercise position is similar to the superman (pages 190-191). Quality supervision is vital. Be doubly sure that your client maintains the neutral position at all times during this exercise and is performing abdominal hollowing. Place a bench or stool in front of the machine, level with your client's shoulders. He should place his hands on the stool in a push-up position, with his legs locked onto the machine pads. He lifts first one hand and then both hands from the stool, placing his arms by his sides. Have him perform this action 10 times, resting his arms on the stool between each movement.

Once he can perform this action in a controlled manner, add spinal extension. He should begin in the neutral position (with or without stool support), move into extension, lifting the shoulders about 2-3 inches (5-8 cm) above the hip only, then back to neutral, and finally down into flexion. Avoid full inner-range extension, to reduce loading on the lumbar facet joints.

Note that *this action can injure an individual with poor back stability.* At the beginning of the movement, if the abdominal muscles are relaxed, the pelvis will anteriorly tilt and the lumbar spine hyperextend, compressing the lumbar facet joints without sufficient intra-abdominal pressure to reduce the loading. Back stability and good alignment control are essential prerequisites for performing this exercise.

Seated Rowing

GOAL *To strengthen scapular retractors (middle trapezius, lower trapezius, serratus anterior) and glenohumeral extensors (triceps)—bilateral.*

Instruct your client to perform this exercise with her knees bent, in order to relax the hamstrings and allow the pelvis to anteriorly tilt sufficiently for her lumbar spine to remain in neutral position. The action is upper arm extension, keeping the elbows in to the sides of the body. The scapulae 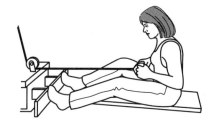 should adduct, and the thoracic spine extend in the sternal lift action (chapter 7). When lowering the weight, she should not allow it to pull the thoracic spine into flexion.

Single Arm Pulley Row

GOAL *Strengthens scapular retractors and shoulder extensors (as in seated rowing)—unilateral.*

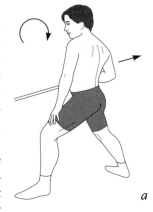

Because this exercise combines back extension and rotation with shoulder extension, it offers a significant challenge to the stabilizing system of the back. Have your client stand in a lunge position to the left of the pulley, with the left foot forward and the D handle of the low pulley gripped in the right hand. He should place his left hand on the left knee for support and angle his body forward (trunk on hip) at 45°. He then pulls the right arm into extension at the shoulder—and, as the pulley hand approaches his chest, he slightly rotates his trunk to the right and extends the thoracic spine (a) (sternal lift action, see chapter 7). Using a low pulley position (pulley at mid-shin level) requires the exerciser to lean over slightly, increasing the workload on the spinal extensors (b). This is suitable only where alignment is good and the individual can keep his spine straight throughout the action. Placing the pulley at waist height negates the requirement to lean forward, taking the workload off the spinal extensors and reducing leverage on the spine. Use the waist-high position if your client's alignment is poor.

a

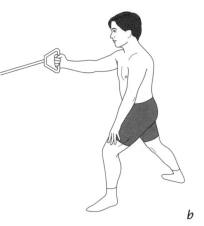

b

Low Pulley Spinal Rotation

GOAL *Strengthens oblique abdominals.*

One can perform spinal rotation exercises in lying, sitting, or standing positions. For the **lying** exercise (a), have your client assume a half-crook lying position perpendicular to the direction of pull, flexing the leg closer to the pulley. Attach the cable of the pulley to

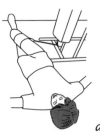

a

continued

Low Pulley Spinal Rotation, continued

the flexed knee with a leather or webbing strap. The action is to rotate the spine so that the bent knee passes over the straight leg and onto the floor.

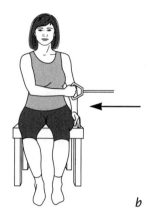

In the **sitting** position (b), your client sits on a stool, facing perpendicular to the pulley, with her left side about 18 inches (0.5 m) from the pulley. She should flex her right arm 90° at the elbow, holding it across her body. After adjusting the level of the lower pulley so that it is level with her elbow, she should grip the D handle of the pulley with her right hand. The action is to rotate her trunk to the right, keeping her hips,

b

legs, and arm immobile so the weight of the pulley unit is lifted by the trunk action alone.

The **standing** exercise is similar to the sitting. She again adjusts the pulley to elbow level and folds the outer arm across her body, her feet apart to maintain a wide base of support.

Rotary Torso Machine

GOAL *To strengthen oblique abdominals while avoiding end-range movements.*

Position the rotation lock to allow full rotation range but *not* to overstretch the spine. If rotation is painful or the range is limited, set the lock of the machine to avoid the painful end-range position. The action is a smooth rotation into full muscular inner range. Have your client hold the position and then slowly release it, avoiding the temptation to drop the weights rapidly and spin the machine. Reset the machine for the opposite rotation, remembering that range and strength are not necessarily symmetrical.

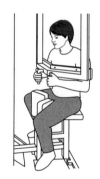

Remember also that the full inner-range position into which an individual's muscles can pull (*physiological* inner range) is generally less than the full inner range into which he can be taken passively (*anatomical* inner range). As long as the motion is smooth and not too fast, your client is in no danger of overly stressing the facet joints of the spine during this exercise. If the motion is too rapid, however, the momentum of the machine can take the spine past physiological inner range and into anatomical inner range, loading the facet joints unnecessarily.

Abdominal Machine

GOAL *Strengthens the rectus abdominis.*

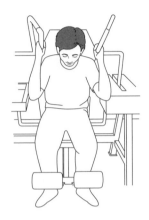

Several abdominal machines are available on the market, but most provide resistance to trunk flexion, emphasizing the supraumbilical portion of the rectus abdominis. Some provide additional resistance for the hip flexors working the infraumbilical portion of rectus abdominis as well. If possible, align the pivot of the machine with the center or lower portion of the lumbar spine rather than the hips. It is important that the rectus abdominis does not bulge outward or "bowstring" during the action, but abdominal hollowing (practiced in *all* these exercises) will alleviate this potential problem. Have your client grip the machine arms, holding his elbows in throughout the action. Instruct him to "roll into flexion," keeping his back on the backrest and avoiding the tendency to lean forward. The movement begins by pulling the sternum *down* rather than *forward*. The eccentric component of the movement is important, so lowering the weight has to be slow and controlled.

Trunk Flexion With High Pulley (Pulley Crunch)

GOAL *Strengthens the rectus abdominis.*

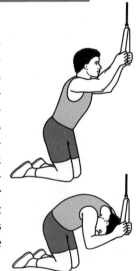

Instruct your client either to kneel (2-point kneeling) or to sit, with his back to the machine, holding the D handle of the machine in both hands behind or in front of the neck (either is correct—the client should choose the most comfortable position). He should shuffle forward until he has taken up the slack in the machine cable. The action is to *flex the trunk alone* rather than the trunk on the hip (hip hinging), with the movement pointing the head downward toward the knees rather than forward in front of the knees. The action must be slow and controlled. Very little movement is available, so it is essential that the machine cable is tight before the action begins.

Free Weight Exercises

In the context of a back stability program, free weights are only for people whose bodies have heavy demands for strength and speed—generally, individuals who perform either medium or heavy manual handling on their jobs, or who are involved in strenuous sports. Free weights are also helpful in late-stage rehabilitation because of the complexity of skills they require (as compared with machine weights).

It is best if, before beginning this stage, your clients have mastered the machine weight exercises just described, as those exercises help build the strength needed in these more complex free weight movements. They must do the exercises in this section only under strict supervision until they have perfected the actions. Give special consideration to clients younger than 18 or older than 60 years of age because their skeletons and joint structures are generally more prone to injury that those of other people. These individuals should exercise only under the supervision of a physical therapist or trainer who is specially trained to teach these groups.

> **KEY POINT:** Individuals must demonstrate good stability, segmental control, and whole-body alignment before beginning late-stage rehabilitation exercises.

Special Concerns Regarding Free Weights

Because free weight exercises combine both *speed* and *weight*, they expose the body to high levels of **momentum** (the product of mass × velocity). It's easy to stop a fast-moving arm if you have a pencil in your hand; but an arm moving at the same speed with a 20-pound weight in the hand can end up with torn tissues if the movement is not controlled. It is important that your sports-oriented clients—whether they swing objects such as racquets, or move their bodies quickly—learn to control momentum forces. The same is true for clients involved in moving or lifting heavy objects on the job.

Before allowing individuals to begin free weight exercises, establish the following prerequisites and ground rules:

• Your clients must have **good stability and alignment.** They must be able to maintain a neutral spinal position against limb resistance, as illustrated by good performance on the heel slide action (chapter 8, page 170). They must be able to maintain good alignment throughout the free weight-training program, keeping their lumbar spines in or near the neutral position at all times—the thoracic spine should be at its optimal position for each client, with shoulders held back comfortably (but not rigidly braced) and the chin held in.

- They must have **good stability endurance.** They should be able to perform 10 repetitions of each of the exercises in chapter 4, holding each rep for 10 seconds.

- They should have **mastered all the machine weight exercises** in the previous section of this chapter.

- They must **warm up and stretch thoroughly before** each weight session. First, they should lightly exercise (treadmill, stationary bike, etc.) till they just begin to sweat. Second, they should perform comprehensive stretching exercises that will take every major joint (hip, knee, shoulder, and spine) through its full range of motion. Third, they should rehearse each exercise by performing the first set at a light weight before adding further resistance.

- They must **stretch adequately after** each weight-lifting session.

- At the beginning, a **qualified trainer** should supervise all free weight exercises, until both client and trainer are satisfied that the exercise technique is good.

- Within the context of a back stability program, your clients should perform all free weight exercises **progressively**—first using light weights, then taking a rest period, then progressing to medium weights, another rest period, and finally heavy weights.

- Free weight exercises as part of a stability program **are not competitive;** they are intended to progressively develop your clients' abilities to perform work against a resistance at speed. Clients should not compete with each other to see who can lift the most weight.

Basic Free Weight Exercises

For best results, have your clients go through all the following exercises in a single session. These exercises are appropriate for most individuals who fulfill the preliminary requirements just described. All the movements should be slow and well controlled. In the next section, I will describe more advanced exercises for people who need a great deal of "explosive power."

Remember that the exercises are designed to build adequate strength, not bulk. Refer to Baechle (1994) for more detailed descriptions of the teaching points for these exercises. Because free weight exercises require more balance and coordination than do machine exercises, less weight should be used. Prescribe about 10-12 repetitions for each exercise, using a final weight that is comfortable for that number of reps (i.e., if the individual can perform 20 repetitions, the weight is too light; if he/she can perform only 5 reps, it is too heavy). For each exercise, your client should perform 2 or 3 sets of 10-12 repetitions: use a moderate weight (perhaps half the final weight) for the first set, three-fourths the final weight for the second, and the full weight only during the third set. In this way, the muscles gradually become accustomed to handling the weight. Your clients should rest after each set until their breathing rates and heart rates return to normal—never let them start a fresh set while their hearts are pounding or they are out of breath. Explain to your more impatient clients that this type of training is designed to "encourage" strength adaptation, not to "force" it. Training should be slow and controlled rather than fast and furious.

Prescribe 2 or 3 sets for each exercise, three sessions per week, skipping at least one day between sessions. After two weeks, they may increase the target weight, again according to how much they can lift comfortably. Let them follow this program—2 or 3 sets of 10-12 reps, three sessions/week—for a period of at least 16 weeks, never increasing the weights to the point where they feel exhausted.

Remember that exercises described for just one side should be done on both sides, and that the instructions for the side not described are, of course, the mirror image of the instructions given.

Lying Barbell Row

GOAL *To strengthen shoulder retractors and increase thoracic spine extension (correct kyphotic posture).*

Instruct your client to lie prone on top of a gym bench, with a light barbell (about 22.5-32.5 lb., or 10-15 kg) beneath the bench. She should grip the barbell at arm's length and lift it until it touches the underside of the bench. She may hold her elbows either close to the sides of her chest or with arms abducted to 90°—the narrow position places greater work on the latissimus dorsi, while the wider grip emphasizes the posterior deltoids and scapular stabilizers.

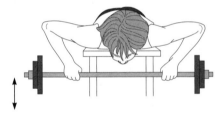

Dumbbell Row

GOAL *Helps correct asymmetry between the shoulder retractors (middle and lower trapezius, serratus anterior).*

You can recognize asymmetry by your client's inability to lift the same amount of weight, or to perform the same number of repetitions, with each arm. Have your client assume the half-kneeling position on a gym bench, his right arm and right knee on the bench and his left leg straight

continued

Dumbbell Row, continued

with his left foot on the ground. He should grip a dumbbell (whatever weight feels comfortable to him) with his left hand, then pull (lift) it toward him, brushing the side of his body with his elbow. He should stop the movement when the dumbbell approaches his chest. As he pulls the upper arm into extension, the scapula is adducted; he should hold the inner-range position for 2-3 seconds before lowering the weight.

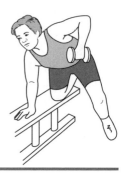

Good Morning

GOAL *Works the spinal extensors statically and the hip extensors dynamically.*

This is basically a hip hinge action (several variations are in chapter 4) performed with a weight. Instruct your client to stand with her feet just wider than shoulder-width apart. Her knees should be unlocked to relax the hamstrings slightly and allow free pelvic tilt. With a light barbell (about 22.5 lb., or 10 kg) across her shoulders, she should tilt her pelvis anteriorly (always maintaining the alignment of the spine to the pelvis) so that her trunk angles forward to 45°. Watch carefully to be sure she

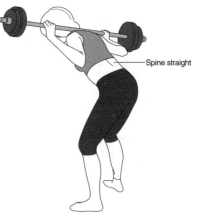

Spine straight

does not allow her spine to flex, moving the axis of rotation from the hip joint to the midlumbar spine—this stresses the spine considerably and can increase intradiscal pressure sufficiently to cause severe injury.

Squat

GOAL *Teaches correct spinal alignment and strengthens the quadriceps, hamstrings, and gluteals.*

Have your client practice the correct form and movement using a light wooden pole (e.g., broom handle) until she has perfected the technique. The beginning weight should be 10-30% of body weight, depending on body build—stronger clients can use the larger value. Instruct your cli-

continued

Squat, continued

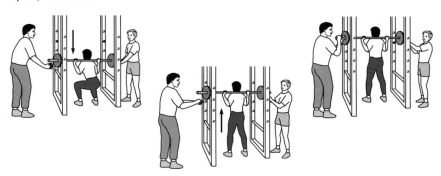

ent always to use a squat rack, so she can take the bar in the standing position. Her feet should be shoulder-width apart, toes turned out slightly. She should step under the bar, her hips directly under her shoulders, and, gripping the bar with hands slightly wider than shoulder width, place it across the back of her shoulders (over the posterior deltoids and trapezius). She should perform a sternal lift action and straighten both legs to lift the bar off the rack—then take a small step backward to clear the bar from the rack.

Throughout the movement, your client should look up and keep her spine nearly vertical. The action is to flex hips and knees simultaneously, keeping the weight of the bar over the center of the foot rather than the toes. Instruct her to lower the bar under control until her thighs are parallel to the ground. After a momentary pause in this lower position to assist balance *(but no bounce!)*, she reverses her actions to lift the bar. Watch to be sure her upward movement is controlled (no increase in speed toward the end of the action) and her knees stay over the foot rather than moving apart or together. Table 9.1 lists common errors associated with the squat.

Table 9.1   Common Errors When Performing a Squat

Error	Technique modification
Knees come inward ("knock-kneed" position).	Foot may be hyperpronating; consider more supportive footwear. Practice a knee-bend position onto a bench in front of a mirror.
Knees stay behind feet throughout movement.	Check if dorsiflexion range is limited in the ankle, and use a wooden block beneath the heels. Practice sitting onto a bench, pressing the knee forward onto the instructor's hand.

continued

Squat, continued

Table 9.1 *(continued)*

Error	Technique modification
Back angles too far forward.	Press the knee forward, and aim to keep the spine more vertically aligned. Practice the basic squat motion side-on to a mirror.
Spine flexes in thoracic region.	Ensure that adequate thoracic extension range is available, and practice the sternal lift motion in isolation. Strengthen the shoulder retractors and stretch the shoulder protractors (page 161).
Anterior pelvic tilt is exaggerated and lumbar lordosis increases.	Strengthen the abdominal muscles, and check for tightness in the hip flexors (chapter 7, pages 144-150). Practice back flattening (chapter 7, page 149) against a wall.
Heel lifts.	Ensure that the weight of the bar is taken through the center of the foot, not through the toes. Check for adequate dorsiflexion range in the ankle, and use a wooden block beneath the heel.
Bar dips to one side.	Practice the squat in front of a mirror, and use a horizontal line drawn on the mirror to line up the reflection of the barbell.
Bouncing in the low position.	Practice squatting onto a bench or stool, lowering gradually into the final position.

Barbell Lunge

GOAL *Helps improve spinal alignment and leg power, but with less spinal compression than in a squat.*

The start position is with the bar across the shoulders as for the squat. Because only one leg leads the movement, less weight (less than half) is used than in a squat—and so less spinal compression is created. Have your client stand with feet shoulder-width apart, the feet marking the end of an imaginary rectangle on the floor in front of him (shoulder-width wide and twice shoulder-width long). As in the squat, he should perform a sternal lift action while maintaining spinal alignment. Instruct him to step directly forward with the right leg (as though placing his

continued

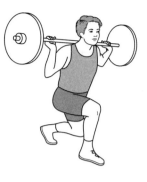

Barbell Lunge, continued

foot along the long edge of the rectangle), then bend his knees so that the knee of the leading leg obscures the foot and that of the trailing leg moves toward the ground, stopping when it is 2-4 inches (5-10 cm) above the floor. The side of the trailing knee should be 6-14 inches (15-35 cm) from the inner edge of the heel of the leading foot. To stand up again, he pushes off the leading leg, bringing the leading foot back to its shoulder-width start position.

The movement must not involve "falling" into the lower position or "jumping" into the upright position. Throughout the movement, your client should look up and forward, and the bar should remain horizontal.

Free Weight Exercises for Explosive Power

Because of unusually heavy demands at work or in strenuous sport activities, some individuals require a high degree of *explosive* strength (i.e., movement against a resistance [the weight] performed at speed [rapid resisted movements]).

A variety of free weight exercises can help develop explosive power in the late stages of a sport-specific or workplace-specific back stability program. In order to perform these exercises, your clients must have progressed through the full back stability program and have good segmental control and spinal alignment. They should have mastered the machine exercises and basic free weight exercises in the previous section of this chapter. Have them rehearse all of the power movements using a wooden pole.

Although you should still prescribe 2 or 3 sets of 10-12 reps, the first set should be with an empty bar to be doubly sure that the technique is correct and to train the muscles in the correct movements. *Your primary guide for subsequent sets must be spinal alignment rather than the amount of weight the client can comfortably lift.* If alignment is degraded, stop the exercise and reduce the weight, even if the client feels the resulting weight is "too light." Remember: the aim here is rehabilitation, not competitive weight lifting or body sculpting.

KEY POINT: For advanced free weight exercises, determine the amount of weight not according to how much your client can lift—rather, by how much your client can lift *and still maintain correct alignment of the spine.*

Hang Clean

GOAL *Stage I power training.*

Have your client begin with the barbell (held with hands pronated) resting on the middle of the thighs. For this exercise you should hand the bar to your client, who is already in the basic position illustrated by (a). Her body should be angled forward (30-45°) at the hips, and her spine straight. Knees and hips should be flexed, ankles dorsiflexed. The action is divided into two phases: the *upward movement* and the *catch*. During the *upward movement*, have your client hold her trunk erect and lift the bar explosively in a single "jump" action, extending the hips and knees and plantarflexing the ankles, without allowing her feet to come off the ground. Her shoulders should stay directly over the bar, and the path of the bar should be as close to the body as possible. At the point of maximum plantarflexion of the ankle, her shoulders will begin to shrug to continue the upward path of the bar (b).

During the *catch* phase, which follows the shoulder shrug as a continuous motion, the client maintains the upward movement by flexing her arms. The elbows drop under the bar, forcing the wrists into extension to allow the bar to rest on the now horizontal palms (c). The elbows point directly forward, and the bar rests over the anterior aspect of the shoulders. As the bar touches the shoulders, your client should slightly flex her knees and hips to absorb shock and prevent a sudden jolt of the bar as she catches it on her shoulders.

Instruct your client to lower the bar all the way to the ground, at first simply by reversing her earlier actions—she dips beneath the bar by bending her knees slightly, then allows her elbows to drop, with the bar staying close to the body as it is lowered. Her knees should bend so her body is not pulled into spinal flexion as the bar approaches the ground.

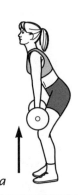
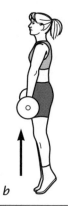
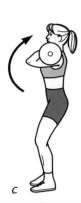

a   *b*   *c*

Power Clean

GOAL *Stage II power training.*

The power clean is a progression from the hang clean, with your client now lifting the weight from the floor rather than from the thighs. The barbell rests either on the floor or on two racks about 10-20 inches (25-50 cm) high. Instruct your client to stand with feet shoulder-width apart and knees inside the arms, feet flat and turned out slightly. It is important with this exercise that your client wears supportive training shoes—preferably a weight-lifting boot or high-cut cross-training shoes with broad, stable heels.

Your client should grasp the bar with hands slightly wider than shoulder-width apart, arms straight. She should squat down so that her shins are almost in contact with the bar, her knees over the center of her feet, her shoulders over or slightly in front of the bar (a). A common error with this movement is to get closer to the bar by flexing the spine, using only limited knee and hip flexion. *This markedly increases the stress on the spine and must be avoided.* The lift consists of three uninterrupted phases: (1) Instruct your client to extend her knees and move her hips forward as she raises her shoulders. Her shins should stay back (a common error with novices is to hit the knees with the bar), always maintaining the alignment of her back. The line of the bar's movement should be vertical, with her heels staying on the ground and the bar passing close to her body (b). Her shoulders should stay back, either over or slightly in front of the bar, and she should position her head to look straight ahead or slightly up. (2) For the "scoop," she drives her hips forward, keeping her shoulders over the bar and her elbows fully extended. The trunk is nearly vertical at this stage (c). This movement brings the bar to the midpoint of the thighs. (3) The exercise continues here as if it were the hang clean, through the upward movement and catch phases of that exercise (see illustrations for hang clean, previous page).

The action is one of continuous movement, with no significant pauses between sections. Although the bar maintains its momentum, your client should never lose control of the movement. She should lower the bar in a vertical path, bending her knees to prevent her spine from being pulled into flexion.

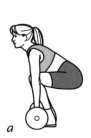
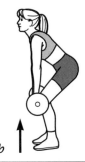
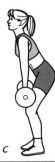

a *b* *c*

Dead Lift

GOAL *To improve back and hip strength, and add power for lifting.*

The exercise begins with the bar on the floor (novices may use low racks at first, until they gain control through the full range of the exercise). Your client should stand with feet flat on the floor (heels must not lift) and shoulder-width apart, knees inside the arms, gripping the bar with hands pronated and slightly wider than shoulder-width apart, elbows pointing out to the sides. (Some athletes use an alternate grip, with one forearm pronated and the other supinated, i.e., knuckles down. If your client finds this grip more comfortable, by all means let him use it— only suggest that he alternate which hand is pronated and which supinated.) Have him position the bar over the balls of his feet, almost touching the shins, with his shoulders over or slightly ahead of the bar and his spine aligned in its neutral position (a).

The movement begins by extending the knees and driving the hips forward. At the same time, your client raises his shoulders so that the alignment of his back remains unchanged. The path of the bar is initially vertical, and it is held close to the body at all times (b). The elbows must not bend, as that will cause a loss of power, and the shoulders should stay over or slightly in front of the bar. The head should be placed so that your client looks forward. Feet should remain flat. As the knees approach full extension, the back begins to move on the hip, maintaining spinal alignment (c). Have your client lower the bar with a squat motion, still maintaining the spine erect, keeping the bar close to the shins.

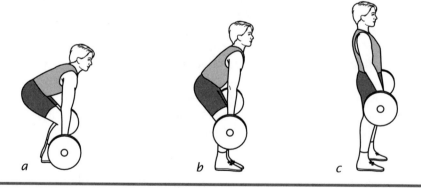

a   *b*   *c*

USING PLYOMETRICS TO TRAIN FOR POWER AND SPEED

For most recreational athletes, almost any kind of training with more rapid movements (such as those in the free weight exercises) will suffice to improve speed. For clients who participate in higher levels of sports competition, however, or who simply want greater fitness gains than they have obtained after mastering everything in this book through chapter 8, proceed to the following plyometric exercises. These exercises can boost both reaction time and response time to high levels.

There is no simplistic formula to help you decide, in consultation with your clients, whether they should do the exercises in this section in addition to the weight-training work just described, or instead of the weight-training exercises. Together, you must weigh your clients' precise needs and goals. The main considerations will probably center around your clients' needs either for especially quick, strong reactions (e.g., hockey goalies or rodeo athletes), or for simple strength that must be explosive, but not necessarily blinding in its speed (e.g., football players or iron workers). If your client has the time and inclination, prescribe both kinds of exercise; if he has neither, but still wants to do more advanced work, choose either the weight training or the plyometrics.

In order for you to understand the physiology behind the exercises, I need to present a bit of theoretical background. First, a few definitions: **Power** is the rate at which work is performed (work/time). Within the context of sports, Kent (1994) defined power as the ability to transform physical energy into force at a fast rate. **Speed** is simply the rate of movement. **Reaction time** is the time from the presentation of a stimulus to the initiation of a response. In terms of muscle work for stabilization, muscle reaction time is the time between the onset of a passive movement that disrupts stability and the initiation of muscle contraction to restabilize the joint. **Response time** combines both reaction time and movement time, the latter dependent on a variety of factors such as energy availability, nerve conduction, and actin/myosin coupling. *Good muscle reaction time is vital to improving joint stability.* Following ligamentous injury, for example, it is the reaction time of the supporting peroneus muscles that is the deciding factor for the return of full function—not just the strength of the muscles (Freeman et al. 1965; Konradsen and Ravn 1990). And following knee injury, the important factor for rehabilitation is the reaction time of the hamstring muscles to resist anterior displacement of the tibia—not the strength of those muscles (Beard et al. 1994).

The **stretch-shorten cycle** is important for anyone who trains for power and speed. Normally, the muscle supplies force through purely chemical means as actin and myosin filaments bond to cause the muscle to shorten. When an eccentric contraction (controlled lengthening) precedes a concentric action, however, force increases dramatically. Observe how a batter always swings his arms back immediately before swinging at a baseball. Or compare a squat jump (jumping from a static squatting position) with a countermovement jump (standing, dropping into a squat position, and then jumping). The height gained with the latter is greater than that from the former. Enoka (1988) measured average heights of 32.4 cm for squat jumps, but 36.4 cm for countermovement jumps—more than 12% greater. The increased height comes from two sources: release of stored elastic energy, and additional chemical energy through a preload effect.

> **KEY POINT:** In a **countermovement,** the extra energy gained relative to a standard movement comes from the release of stored *elastic energy* within the muscle, and from the *preload* effect.

Elastic energy results from passive stretching of the elastic components of the muscle. The muscle membranes (endomysium, epimysium, etc.) are noncontractile, but they are elastic and will recoil when released from a stretch, as will muscle tendons. The combined recoil of membranes and tendons provides a significant amount of energy.

It takes time for actin and myosin coupling to occur. Chemical energy increases in a countermovement because, when the muscle is contracted eccentrically before it is contracted concentrically, the additional time permits more coupling—which leads to release of more chemical energy. Providing extra time to allow chemical reactions to occur creates the **preload effect.** Think of elastic energy as the muscle's springing back or recoiling like an elastic band—it is passive, and physical; whereas preload is like giving the muscle a running start on the chemical processes that lead to earlier contraction—it is active, and chemical.

Three factors are important to energy release during concentric-eccentric coupling (Enoka 1988):

1. **Time.** If there is a delay between stretching the muscle and concentric contraction, some of the stored energy is dissipated. During the delay, actin and myosin filaments become detached and reattach farther along the muscle fiber under less stretch.

2. **Magnitude.** If the stretch magnitude is too great, fewer crossbridges are able to remain attached, and less elastic energy is available.

3. **Velocity.** A more rapid stretch (greater velocity) creates more elastic energy.

To create maximum power with concentric-eccentric coupling, an individual must be warmed up; and a rapid eccentric movement must be followed immediately by a rapid concentric movement with *no rest between the two phases.* Any standard exercise *can* be performed in this way, and the exercises created are known as **plyometrics.** Yet not all exercises *should* be included in a plyometric workout since leverage forces and momentum acting on the spine can be dangerous: beware especially of rapid end-range motion on the spine and long lever movements.

Before You Start

Before progressing to the following plyometric exercises, your clients must

- demonstrate good basic stability—able to perform the heel slide exercise (chapter 8, page 170) 10 times, and in general to perform adequately the exercises in chapter 4;

- demonstrate good power and control in the trunk—able to perform gym ball exercises, including the superman (chapter 8, page 190) and bridge (chapter 8, page 191); and

- have good overall general fitness—demonstrated by regular, moderate-to-intense exercise over the previous six to eight weeks. The exercise intensity should have been sufficient to raise the heart rate above 100 beats per minute. Each exercise session should have lasted for a minimum of 20 continuous minutes, with three periods of exercise per week.

Plyometric Exercises

A number of exercises are useful. Be certain that your clients are supervised during all of them until both subjects and trainers are satisfied that your clients have learned the proper technique. Have your clients perform each exercise (for both right and left sides if it is asymmetrical) a maximum of 20 times per session, stopping earlier if they lose alignment or abdominal hollowing. They should try from one to three sessions per week for at least eight weeks, gradually increasing the speed of their movements as they are able. After the eight-week period, your clients may stop using plyometrics unless they are competitive athletes who require explosive strength to aid performance—in which case their strength coaches should prescribe the advanced plyometric exercises, tailoring them to the athletes' particular sports or events.

Plyometric Side Bend Using a Punching Bag

GOAL *Develops power and speed of the trunk side flexors while maintaining back stability.*

Instruct your client to stand with his left side toward a punching bag, feet shoulder-width apart, with his left arm abducted to 90°. He should flex his trunk to the left and *push* (not hit) the bag with his straight left arm. As the bag swings back, he takes its weight with his straight arm, then side flexes to the right to decelerate the swing of the bag (stopping short of full range!). The left side flexion begins the motion again. The action is reversed with the subject standing with his right side toward the bag.

Plyometric Flexion and Extension Using a Punching Bag

GOAL *Develops power and speed in the trunk flexors and extensors while maintaining back stability.*

Have your client stand facing the punching bag, then push the bag with one or both hands. He should follow the movement through, *using trunk flexion only*, to 45°. He remains in this flexed position, and, as the bag swings back, he takes the bag with his arms straight (but unlocked) and flexes the arms, extending his trunk minimally and transferring his body weight to his back foot to cushion the momentum of the moving bag.

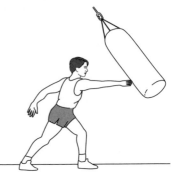

Twist and Throw With Medicine Ball

GOAL *Develops power and speed of the trunk rotators while maintaining back stability.*

Your client should stand in an aligned posture, with stabilized trunk and minimal abdominal hollowing. A training partner, facing in the same direction as your client, stands about three feet to her right, holding a medicine ball. While your client rotates her trunk to the right, her partner throws the medicine ball to her. As she catches the ball, she should rotate to the left, prestretching the oblique abdominals. She stops the movement short of full range, rotates back to the right, and throws the ball back to her partner.

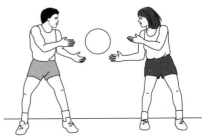

Medicine Ball Trunk Curl

GOAL *Develops power and speed in the trunk flexors while maintaining back stability.*

This exercise is a modification of the trunk curl (chapter 6, page 126). Instruct both your client and his training partner to lie on a mat with

continued

Medicine Ball Trunk Curl, continued

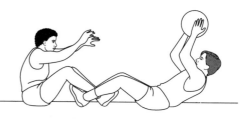

their knees bent (crook lying), such that their ankles are almost touching. They should then raise their trunks (without significantly moving their legs) to a stable upright position. The training partner throws a medicine ball to your client, who catches it while in the upright position, holding it close to his chest, but then moves back into the lower trunk curl position. He should stop the movement short of full range (his back should not touch the ground), then "bounce" back with a concentric trunk curl and throw the ball back to his partner. Increase the range of the curling action by having your client lie over a cushion—this allows the trunk to move into extension before moving into flexion. Be sure that movement stops short of full range *in each direction* in order to reduce joint loading.

Leg Raise Throw

GOAL *To develop power and speed in the lower abdominals.*

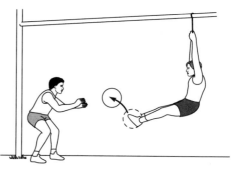

Make sure your client can easily perform the wall bar hanging leg raise (page 129) before attempting this movement. Your client should hang from a gymnasium beam with a ball beneath him. Instruct him to grip the ball between both feet, then flex his hips and spine to throw the ball forward to a waiting partner. The partner places the ball back between your client's feet while the hips are still flexed to 90°. Your client then lowers his legs to prestretch the lower abdominals before repeating the movement.

SUMMARY

- It is imperative that individuals be able to consistently hollow their abdomens, contract their multifidus muscles at will, and maintain neutral position before they attempt these exercises.

- After (and only after) your client has attained basic back stability using exercises presented earlier in this book, he/she can progress to using (1) machine exercises and/or (2) plyometric exercises, each of which can further stabilize the back and help prevent future injury.
- Basic free weight exercises are useful for people whose jobs or sport activities demand greater back stability than that created by the earlier exercises.
- Advanced free weight exercises are appropriate for those whose jobs or sport activities are extremely demanding and require "explosive strength."
- Plyometric exercises are particularly useful for individuals who need *very fast* reaction times along with strength in their movements.
- Because the material in this chapter is specifically designed for individuals with a history of low back pain, the exercises may differ from those you might prescribe for other individuals.

Putting It
All Together

Although chapters 1 through 9 provide everything you really need to know in order to prescribe a very effective back stability program for virtually any client, I have summarized some ideas in chapter 10 ("Building a Back Stability Program for Your Client") that should help you synthesize the theoretical and practical material more easily. In chapter 10, you'll learn more about how to deal with pain since you generally will need to take care of that before even attempting to prescribe exercises. And I provide general tips about how to decide which exercises to prescribe for whom. Possibly the most helpful part of this chapter is the four case histories, which help you understand how to deal with four different kinds of client, from your first meeting until you discharge them.

Chapter 11, "Preventing Back Injuries and Reinjuries," advocates a more proactive approach to dealing with your clients' daily activities. It is very common for people to reinjure themselves by lifting objects they had no business lifting, or by lifting them in the wrong way. Some therapists merely hand clients a pamphlet that describes proper lifting procedures, but most clients do not take written material alone very seriously. Chapter 11 shows you how to teach your clients to avoid reinjury, with the suggestion that you actually do a bit of role-playing in order to help your clients *internalize* the theoretical principles.

10

Building a Back Stability Program for Your Client

We have come full circle from the preface and seen how the three components of muscle imbalance—correction of segmental control, shortening and strengthening lax muscles, and lengthening tight muscles—combine to produce back stability. Although there is a great deal of highly varied material in previous chapters, you should nevertheless find it rather easy to tailor a unique back stability program to each client, taking these three components into account as they are needed for each individual. It is largely a question of (1) assessing where the problems lie and (2) prescribing appropriate exercises to correct the problems. Yet before you even think about a back stability program for a given individual, make sure that you should be treating the individual in the first place.

PRELIMINARY ASSESSMENT OF YOUR CLIENT

Especially for individuals who have experienced serious cardiovascular illness, you must decide whether exercise is appropriate at all. It is rare, but occasionally you may see someone whose general health is in such a state that the slightest additional stress could be catastrophic. If you have any doubts about an individual, be sure to have him or her obtain clearance through a medical doctor before proceeding with therapy. Note also that, although a back stability program is generally suitable for even the very unfit, it is contraindicated in some cases where people are not able to practice it correctly. If hypertensive individuals cannot be taught to hollow without holding their breath, for example, then hollowing is clearly contraindicated. And advanced exercises using weights are contraindicated in cases of reduced bone density.

Pain

If clients are in pain when they first come to you, manage the pain *before* proceeding with any muscle training. If you are qualified to treat the pain, then apply whatever treatments you deem appropriate. If you are not qualified, refer clients to someone who is and work jointly with that therapist. Pain can inhibit muscle contraction and can affect alignment by making people take up positions that are less painful, but that reinforce poor alignment. It is certainly true that back stability exercise can lead to significant pain relief (e.g., multifidus training can release back spasms), but such activities work best when used as an adjunct to pain-relieving treatments.

Where pain is extreme, elimination of the pain may become the *primary* aim of treatment. Pain that occurs through muscle spasm, or through trigger points in tight muscles, may be relieved by treatments that reduce muscle tone—various physical therapy treatments, manual therapy, and/or stretching. See Norris (1999) for details of these types of treatment.

Where pain is the result of persistent overstress on a hypermobile segment, focus initial treatments on segmental control and stability. You may have to create stability passively at first (through taping or splinting), until your client has gained sufficient control of the muscular stabilizing system.

Diagnostic Triage

Diagnostic triage categorizes low back pain into three types: simple back ache; nerve root pain (the nerve root is the "T" junction of the nerve as it joins to the spinal cord—pain from this area indicates compression of the nerve by a spinal disc or other structure); or possibly serious pathology requiring referral to a specialist (Waddell et al. 1997). See "Diagnostic Triage," page 233. I do not generally recommend referral to a specialist for simple back ache, and clients with nerve root compression do not usually require referral *if* their pain resolves within four weeks of its onset. Clients with possibly serious pathology require prompt referral, while those with likely **cauda equina syndrome** (involving a group of fine nerves at the base of the spinal cord) require *immediate* referral. For individuals with simple back ache or nerve root compression, you generally can begin back stability exercises immediately (with or without other physical therapy treatment). Those with serious pathology, however, may require surgical intervention before you begin back stability exercise, but please note the discussion in chapter 1, page 6, concerning the appropriateness of surgery on low back pain. Back stability exercise is a necessity as follow-up therapy for those with a previous history of back pain but no current pain, and as a preventive therapy for clients with no history of back pain (table 10.1).

Diagnostic Triage

Diagnostic triage is the differential diagnosis between

1. Simple back pain (nonspecific low back pain—i.e., pain with no specific cause)
2. Nerve root compression
3. Possibly serious spinal pathology (such as bone damage, infection, carcinoma, or pain traveling/referred from the abdomen or gastro/urinary systems)

1. Simple back ache: *specialist referral not required*

Patient aged 20-55 years

Pain restricted to lumbosacral region, buttocks, or thighs

Pain is "mechanical" (i.e., pain changes with and can be relieved by movement)

Patient otherwise in good health (no temperature, nausea/dizziness, weight loss, etc.)

2. Nerve root pain: *specialist referral not generally required within first four weeks, if the pain is resolving*

Unilateral (one side of the body) leg pain that is worse than low back pain

Pain radiates into the foot or toes

Numbness and paresthesia (altered feeling) in the same area as pain

Localized neurological signs (such as reduced tendon jerk and positive nerve tests)

3. Red flags (caution) for possibly serious spinal pathology: *refer promptly to specialist*

Patient under 20 or over 55 years of age

Nonmechanical pain (i.e., pain does not improve with movement)

Thoracic pain

Past history of carcinoma, steroid drugs, or HIV

Patient unwell or has lost weight

Widespread neurological signs

Obvious structural deformity (such as bone displacement after an accident, or a lump which has appeared recently)

Sphincter disturbance (unable to pass water or incontinent)

Gait disturbance (unable to walk correctly)

Saddle anesthesia (no feeling in crotch area between the legs)

Cauda equina syndrome (*refer to specialist immediately—i.e., same day*)

If in doubt, always refer the patient to an orthopedic physical therapist.

Adapted, by permission, from G. Waddell, G. Feder, and M. Lewis, 1997, "Systematic reviews of bed rest and advice to stay active for acute low back pain," *British Journal of General Practice* 47: 647-652.

Table 10.1 Use of Back Stability Exercises

Type of back pain	Back stability exercise
Simple	Begin immediately; continue until fully functional.
Nerve root compression	Begin as pain allows; refer to specialist if no marked progress within four weeks.
Serious pathology	Use back stability exercise after surgical/medical intervention.
Previous back pain now resolved	Use back stability exercise to restore full function.
No history of back pain	Use back stability exercise to reduce risk of developing back pain.

Reprinted, by permission, from G. Waddell, G. Feder, and M. Lewis, 1997, "Systematic reviews of bed rest and advice to stay active for acute low back pain," *British Journal of General Practice* 47: 647-652.

GENERAL PRINCIPLES FOR DESIGNING A STABILITY PROGRAM

There are a few basic principles that apply in every situation:

- If you are not trained to properly diagnose back ailments, proceed no further until you've referred your client to a trained therapist—then work as closely with that therapist as you can, prescribing exercises appropriate to the therapist's diagnoses.
- Remember the general principle that bed rest is counterproductive (see chapter 1). Except in unusual circumstances, get your clients up and performing controlled activities as quickly as possible after an injury.
- Start back stability work as soon as possible after you have determined that such a program is appropriate for an individual. The longer people are unstable, the more likely they are to develop compensatory postures that will need to be retrained.
- Always pay close attention to pain—it can be a very reliable guide. In a careful series of assessments, it can tell you where the problems lie; throughout an individual's program, it can tell you when to stop a given exercise.
- Remember the *principle of specificity:* prescribe specific activities for specific problems/goals. This is why careful assessment is so important. Many therapists have a one-size-fits-all program. I have heard about many unhappy individuals, especially in the United States, who have visited physicians because of back pain—and the way the

doctor "treated" them was to hand them a "back care pamphlet" and instruct them to do all the exercises in it! After reading part I of this book, you know that you must deal with each individual according to his or her precise symptoms.

- Remember the *principle of overload:* if the overload is not great enough, there will be no training effect; your client will merely be engaging in physical activity rather than training. Too great an overload, however, will break down tissue; and since the body cannot adapt sufficiently to match the imposed stress, overuse injury results. Carefully following the exercise programs presented in this book will enable you to achieve a training effect with your clients and to avoid overtraining injuries— a particular danger with those who have experienced low back pain or back injury.

Be sure that you always have a clear vision of your goal for each individual, and of the best path to reach that goal. That path should consider *all systems*—muscle tightness/laxness, posture, strength, flexibility, reaction speed, skill, and even emotional factors. Be careful that you do not fall into the common trap of overemphasizing a single aspect of fitness or rehabilitation. This is especially easy to do when strong-willed, generally knowledgeable clients make it clear that they have a certain problem and they want it fixed in a certain way ("I hurt my back at work, and I need to do some weight training so I can lift boxes again. . ."). *Working one system in isolation can do more harm than good.* Excessive flexibility in relation to strength, for example, may lead to instability of a joint. Individuals with increased strength, but without parallel improvement in muscle reaction speed, may be unable to use their extra strength in functional situations (Konradsen and Ravn 1990). Increases in either strength or flexibility that fail to improve skill may make injury more likely (Tropp et al. 1993).

PARALLEL TRACKS IN DESIGNING A STABILITY PROGRAM

Because the body is a complex unit of closely interconnecting systems, any approach to treatment must be holistic, even if it targets a single system. In training clients for back stability, we constantly intertwine our focuses on correcting segmental control, shortening and strengthening lax muscles, and lengthening tight muscles. The order in which you use these exercises, of course, will depend on your clients' symptoms. You ideally want to pay attention to all these areas at all times. When time constraints require that you teach only one or two exercises, stretches, etc., at a time, simply focus first on the most problematic area. In the accompanying case histories, note how I generally started with just one or two exercises, aiming to solve the most acute problem first.

The following sections provide suggestions for *parallel exercise progressions*. Don't (for example) just look at basic stability, proceed to correct it, and finally go on to other items only after your client can do a great hip hinge. Assess basic stability, deep abdominal control, muscle imbalance, and posture *when you first see a client.* At first, you may need to deal only with the most glaring deficiency, as the case histories illustrate. By your third or fourth treatment session, you generally will want to prescribe appropriate measures to *correct each deficiency at the same time,* working on each "track" during each session, and prescribing home exercises for each area. This is not as time consuming as it sounds, as many of the exercises in this book address several aims at the same time.

Assess Back Stability

Your first task upon seeing a new client is to learn how stable her back is—and, to the degree it is not stable, to determine wherein lies the instability and to begin creating stability through appropriate activities described in chapter 4. *Almost all prescriptive journeys begin in chapter 4.* Your clients should not advance to actual strengthening or even stretching exercises until they have mastered the movements in that chapter.

The best way to begin assessment is with the heel slide (page 170): if the pelvis tilts, your client has an unstable back and you should begin by teaching her abdominal hollowing (chapter 4, page 83). If her pelvis does not move during the heel slide, indicating a degree of stability, begin by teaching your client to control pelvic tilt (chapter 4, page 74) and to assume/maintain the neutral position (chapter 4, page 78), without ignoring abdominal hollowing, of course. She should progress through pelvic tilt actions, to supported hip hinge exercises, and finally to free hip hinge exercises (all in chapter 4).

Once your client demonstrates adequate segmental control by being able to independently control her pelvis and spine, let her progress to the good morning exercise, first without and finally with light barbell weights (chapter 9, page 216).

Assess the Degree of Deep Abdominal Control

Can your client perform abdominal hollowing in the prone kneeling position? If not, follow the instructions under "Teaching Your Clients to Use Abdominal Hollowing" in chapter 4 (page 81), especially the subsection on teaching tips (page 86). Once he has mastered abdominal hollowing in *all* positions, help him gradually build up his strength and endurance till he can perform the movement for 10 reps, 10 seconds each, in the kneeling position. For more advanced abdominal control, he can progress to limb-loading exercises in chapter 8—especially the heel slide (page 170) and leg lowering (page 170).

Assess Muscle Imbalance

For each client, go through all the assessments in chapter 5 under "Assessing Stretched Muscles" (page 103) and under "Assessing Shortened Muscles" (page 106). Then proceed to correct whatever deficiency you find. For stretched or weakened abdominal muscles, for example, prescribe appropriate exercises (look at the "goal" statements) from chapter 6 under "Modifications of Traditional Abdominal Exercises" (page 124) and "Ab Roller Exercises" (page 130). For tightened muscles, refer to "Stretching Target Muscles" in chapter 5 (page 113). If clients have *both* tight muscles *and* an unstable back, I suggest that you begin with stretching exercises—your clients first must learn to *find* the neutral position before they take the second step in doing exercises to help them *maintain* neutral position.

Some clients, especially the elderly, will have chronic muscle tightness that is virtually impossible to cure completely. Yet you are unlikely to meet someone whom you can't help at all—even if you cannot help people achieve optimal posture, you probably can help them move more freely, increase their range of motion, and experience less discomfort.

Assess Posture

Assessing posture goes hand-in-hand with checking muscle balance and can often give the first indication of which muscles may need to be tested for imbalance. Select the procedures under "Basic Postural Assessment" (chapter 7, page 136) that you find most useful given your availability of equipment, and thoroughly assess your client's posture. If you suspect a muscle is lengthened, test its inner-range holding ability (e.g., test the gluteals for lordotic posture); if you think it is tight, use specific tests of muscle length (e.g., for lordotic posture use the Thomas test for tight hip flexors). Then train the muscle accordingly, using inner-range holding for lengthened muscles and static or PNF stretching for tight muscles. See "Principles of Postural Correction" (page 143) and "Posture Types and How to Correct Them" (page 145).

DESIGNING AN ADVANCED STABILITY PROGRAM

After clients have achieved basic back stability, they may wish to press on with more intense work because of heavy physical demands from work or from athletic activities. Chapters 8 and 9 are for such individuals.

In General, Be Specific

The single most important concept is to determine, in close consultation with clients, precisely what their needs/goals are. Does she have to lift 50-pound grain bags all day at work? Is he a tennis player whose body is constantly twisted and exposed to very rapid loads? Is your client a door-man who spends eight hours each day standing up and moving relatively little? Is she a caregiver who must bend over and lift bedridden patients many times a day? Every individual's specific needs will call for specific exercises to strengthen, stretch, increase reaction speed, increase accuracy of movement, or whatever. And there is no way I can suggest sequences of exercises to cover all possibilities.

That is why each exercise is preceded by a "goal" statement. Once you have determined specific goals for a client, select the exercises in chapters 8 and 9 that match those goals. Choosing the exercises is relatively straight-forward. Where you must be very careful is in your exercise prescriptions. I have provided basic guidelines for the exercises in each chapter, either with introductory remarks or with the exercises themselves. But these are no more than guidelines. Carefully monitor your clients as they first per-form any exercise, not only to be sure they are performing the exercises correctly, but also to *be sure they are performing enough reps and using suffi-cient load to challenge their muscles, but not to excessively load them.*

Tips for Designing Weight-Training Programs

In addition to the rather specific instructions I provide for the weight-training exercises, here are a few more strategies you can use to guide your prescriptions of exercises.

The order in which weight-training exercises are performed in a single exercise session is important. In general, have your clients **work large muscle groups first** with *multijoint* exercises, and smaller groups second using *isolation* movements. A multijoint exercise is one that works a num-ber of muscles, including those with a large muscle mass. For example, the bench press works the pectoral muscles and the triceps. Because the triceps are far smaller than the pectorals, they fatigue first and so are the *limiting factor* in the exercise. If the triceps are worked first, fewer bench press movements are possible and the pectoral muscles will not be suffi-ciently challenged.

Another method of combining exercises is to use a **superset** (i.e., to work the muscles on one side of a limb, and then immediately [without a rest] work those on the opposing side). This type of training keeps the blood within a body part, while the individual muscles themselves have some rest. A typical superset routine would involve biceps-triceps-biceps.

One way to provide maximum challenge to muscles is to use **pyramid training.** Have your client perform 12 repetitions with an average weight for the first set, 10 reps with a heavier weight for the second set, and finally 8 reps with the heaviest weight he can manage for the final set. In this way, the muscle is worked maximally, but only when it is thoroughly warmed up. See Norris (1995b) for further details of weight-training programs.

CASE HISTORY

The Overweight Client

A 42-year-old man with a history of persistent back pain, AH worked on a production line. He was about 56 pounds overweight, with marked lordotic posture. The goal of my treatment was first to reduce pain and then to restore postural balance. In the first treatment session, I instructed AH to perform supine lying lumbar flexion, bringing the knees to the chest with overpressure to encourage flexion of the lumbar spine. The principle here was that AH's lordotic posture was placing an excessive extension stress on his low back. The flexion exercise that I used was designed to neutralize this. With repetition (15-25 reps), his low back pain eased. I showed him how to get onto and off the floor without bending and advised him to practice this exercise every two hours of the waking day for two days. I gave AH general advice concerning back care and resting, used standard physical therapy modalities to reduce local pain, and referred him to a dietician to begin a weight-loss program.

By the second treatment session two days later, AH's pain was markedly reduced. I started him on a general aerobic exercise session with his back supported—he used static cycling (seat and handlebar adjusted to minimize back stress) and a ski trainer to perform heart-rate-controlled exercise for 15-20 minutes every other day.

At the second session, I also started AH on stability training, beginning with abdominal hollowing in the 4-point kneeling position and using a webbing belt around his abdomen. Since AH was unable to perform abdominal hollowing correctly, I provided a surface EMG unit to give feedback. It took 40 minutes to re-educate deep abdominal contraction using surface EMG, palpation, and voice encouragement. But since AH was still unable to perform the exercise unaided, I did not yet prescribe abdominal hollowing as a home exercise. AH continued with his back care and aerobic training for two more days.

During his third treatment session, AH was able to perform abdominal hollowing with a 5- to 7-second hold for 3 repetitions. We had to work hard to help him refrain from holding his breath—I encouraged him to count out loud as he performed abdominal hollowing, to show that he was breathing normally.

AH progressed in hollowing his abdomen but found it difficult to control the neutral position of his spine without my feedback. I taught him abdominal hollowing in wall-support standing to allow him to practice at home without having to think about his spine. He used a belt, focusing on pulling his abdominals in and up from the belt. He particularly liked this exercise, as it began to give his abdominal wall a flatter appearance—and, combined with weight loss, AH's physical appearance began to be leaner.

continued

Case History, *continued*

We repeatedly set goals: goals for weight loss, numbers of repetitions performed, holding time of exercises, and heart-rate-monitored exercise.

AH's low back pain had now gone, and he progressed from abdominal hollowing in standing to standing posterior pelvic tilt. Since his cardiopulmonary fitness (measured as heart-rate recovery) had improved with a decline in percent body fat (38% to 30%), I had him increase his aerobic activity. He still used nonweightbearing or partial weightbearing activities in the gymnasium to reduce joint loading, but now he began walking (on grass/gravel with shock absorbing sports shoes) for 15-20 minutes daily.

In an attempt to shorten AH's rectus abdominis, to his standing posterior pelvic tilt I added posterior tilt in the lying position, held for 20-30 seconds (breathing normally). AH had short hip flexors and hamstrings, and he stretched them using the half-kneeling hip flexor stretch and active knee extension. AH built up his stability work with kneeling activities (knee raise, 10 repetitions on each leg, holding for 10 seconds) and began hollowing his abdomen regularly during his walking.

I discharged AH from physical therapy to a personal trainer at a local gymnasium, where he incorporated stability work into a general fitness and weight-loss program.

Points to Note

✔ AH had mechanical back pain brought on by his lordotic posture.

✔ Posture correction began with weight loss.

✔ Because AH was initially unable to perform correct abdominal hollowing, I did not give this as a home exercise.

✔ Surface EMG proved useful in initially teaching abdominal hollowing.

✔ We repeatedly used goal setting.

✔ Since AH liked the standing abdominal hollowing exercise, I used it intensely.

✔ AH used aerobic training to aid general fitness as well as specific back stability.

✔ The back stability program formed a focus for more general lifestyle changes.

✔ When discharged from physical therapy care, AH continued the back stability program in another setting.

CASE HISTORY
Poor Stability in an Athlete

Twenty-six-year-old HC trains daily in a gymnasium, using either weight-training apparatus (40 minutes) plus cardiopulmonary apparatus (20 min-

continued

utes), or step aerobics (60 minutes). One day she complained of low back pain the morning after training. X-ray examination of the low back and pelvic joints showed no abnormality, and blood tests were normal. She was referred to me for physical therapy three months after the onset of pain. Her lumbar spine and sacroiliac joints were unremarkable upon examination, but repeated lumbar extension—especially anterior pelvic tilt—caused pain.

Kinesiological examination (movement analysis) showed poor lumbar stability with overhead movements and with hip extension actions in standing. HC stated that two exercises in particular gave rise to her pain following workouts: standing hip extension on a "multihip" unit that targets the gluteals and repeated overhead pressing actions in standing with an aerobics bar. Examination of these moves showed that her pelvis moved rapidly into anterior tilt and remained in that position throughout the exercises.

In assessing HC's abdominal musculature, I found high tone in the superficial abdominals, with marked muscular definition of the rectus abdominis (the "six pack"). Yet she performed poorly on stability tests, being unable to perform abdominal hollowing in 4-point kneeling while maintaining a neutral lumbar spine. In the heel slide action monitored by a pressure biofeedback unit, HC was unable to perform more than 3 repetitions before her pelvis tilted anteriorly. In 4-point kneeling, leg lifting actions caused marked muscle quivering, demonstrating poor performance.

HC's gross segmental control was also poor—she was unable to perform a controlled hip hinge action. She moved not into spinal flexion (like most people) but into extension, anteriorly tilting her pelvis and hyperextending her lumbar spine.

In her first treatment session, I had her perform supine knee and hip flexion, to press the lumbar spine into flexion. I told her to do these movements at the end of each workout period. I temporarily removed the overhead press and hip extension exercises from her gym program. Following her first two workout periods after the first session, HC noted reduced pain in the mornings.

I used video feedback to show HC her performance in the hip extension and overhead exercises. She was surprised, having been unaware of her lack of alignment. I had HC try to perform abdominal hollowing in 4-point kneeling, and she was able to perform the exercise within 2-3 minutes of being shown the movement. She then used abdominal hollowing in wall-support standing, progressing to free standing after 2 sets of 10 repetitions. She used abdominal hollowing in free standing and free (stool) sitting during her gym workouts, performing a single set with a 30-second hold, breathing normally.

HC progressed quickly (within two weeks) to supine lying heel slide and finally to supine lying foot drop (2 sets, 10 reps, 30-second hold). I prescribed 4-point kneeling knee movements to improve stability control.

continued

Case History, *continued*

By the third treatment session (10 days after beginning treatment), noting that HC was able to perform abdominal hollowing for 10 reps, holding each for 30 seconds, I prescribed the hip hinge action. Initially I had her use controlled pelvic tilt in crook lying. In that same session, she progressed to pelvic tilt in wall-support standing, and finally in free standing. She performed the hip hinge with a stick held along the length of the spine to give feedback about spinal position. Initially she performed the exercise next to a mirror, then without a mirror, then without a stick, and finally with her eyes closed (to overload proprioception). HC had mastered the hip hinge action by her fourth treatment session—at which point I had her perform overhead pressing actions with a stick, and perform hip extensions on the multihip unit with minimal weight. Her goal was to maintain abdominal hollowing and a neutral lumbar alignment throughout the exercise.

I incorporated stability principles of abdominal hollowing (30% max contraction) and neutral lumbar alignment into all of HC's exercise activities.

Points to Note

✔ HC had excellent cosmetic appearance of her abdominal region (superficial abdominals), but poor deep abdominal control.

✔ She was unable to maintain neutral lumbar alignment, even though she had high muscle tone.

✔ I used extensive movement analysis and made a point of observing the exercises that HC practiced in her gym.

✔ She had poor segmental control, moving into extension rather than flexion as is more common.

✔ Video feedback permitted HC to see her alignment. Mirrors and the use of a stick increased feedback.

✔ HC was a regular exerciser and had good body visualization. She was able to pick up new exercise techniques very quickly.

✔ Deep abdominal training and segmental control (hip hinge action) formed the basis of her program.

✔ I waited until after HC was pain free to begin the basic stability program.

Acute Pain

DB, 34 years old, came to me with acute simple low back pain that was localized to the lower lumbar region and minimally referred into the right buttock. The pain was mechanical in nature, made worse by lumbar flexion

continued

and better by lumbar extension. Initially I treated the pain, using physical therapy and lumbar manipulation. Then I had her begin multifidus contractions in left side lying, while I palpated the right multifidus and encouraged her to attempt to "swell" the muscle beneath my fingers. Although unable to perform this action at first, by the end of the second treatment session she was minimally able to contract the multifidus. I had her perform rhythmic stabilizations in left side lying—I placed pressure over her pelvis and shoulder to encourage spinal rotation and instructed DB to resist this motion with slight muscle contraction. As contraction built in intensity, I changed my hand position to resist spinal rotation in the opposite direction. The combination of rhythmic stabilization and isolated multifidus contractions gave substantial pain relief, with pain reducing from 8 to 3 on a subjective scale (10 = most intense pain, 1 = least intense).

In the second treatment session, I introduced abdominal hollowing. As DB lay prone, I instructed her to draw her abdomen in, in an attempt to pull her tummy away from the surface of the treatment table. Since DB was at first unable to perform this action, I used pressure biofeedback, placing the bladder of the biofeedback unit beneath her abdomen just above the top of her pelvis and inflating the bladder sufficiently for DB to feel pressure over the abdomen. I instructed her to draw in her abdomen in an attempt to pull away from the biofeedback unit, thereby reducing the pressure on the bag. I wanted DB to perform the exercise at home, but since she was unable to identify when she was performing abdominal hollowing correctly, I brought her husband into the treatment session and showed him how to assist her. At home, DB placed a folded towel beneath her abdomen in the same position that the biofeedback bladder had occupied. I instructed DB's husband to gently try to slide the towel out from beneath DB's abdomen, while his wife drew in her abdomen sufficiently to take her weight from the towel and permit it to be pulled away. I instructed her to repeat this exercise 3 times daily, performing 10 reps each time.

Once DB was able to perform the hollowing action unaided in the prone lying position, I had her progress to abdominal hollowing in kneeling and sitting positions. While aiding DB in her back stability training, I also instructed her on general back care, with emphasis on correct sitting and resting postures. I also taught her basic lifting techniques for use in the home. She progressed through the early stages of the back stability program using the heel slide, kneeling leg lift, and hip hinge actions. I then referred her to an exercise instructor at a local health club, to perform a general exercise program incorporating back stability principles.

Points to Note

✔ Because DB was in intense pain, I used physical therapy for pain relief at the beginning of her first session, before introducing her to stability exercises later in the session.

continued

Case History, *continued*

✔ On the first day, I began teaching her to control the multifidus, which helped in pain relief.

✔ I used pressure biofeedback and palpation.

✔ I showed a family member how to assist with DB's abdominal hollowing exercises at home.

✔ DB continued her back stability training at a health club, along with general fitness activities.

CASE HISTORY
Patient Unwilling to Exercise

SD was a 53-year-old manual worker in a food company. About 42 pounds overweight, he had marked abdominal sagging and chronic back pain that was localized to the lower lumbar region. His erector spinae muscles were tight and thickened. When standing, SD had a flattened lumbar curve, showing a typical "flatback" posture. Examination of range of movement revealed a lack of lumbar extension, and grossly limited pelvic tilt during forward flexion movements. The pelvis contributed little to forward bending since most forward movement came from the upper lumbar and lower thoracic spine. Examination of SD's lifting techniques showed repeated bending actions with his legs straight, and adoption of poor resting positions with marked spinal flexion. SD had attended his company's manual handling course and even a refresher course, but his line manager confirmed SD's unwillingness to practice correct handling procedures on a regular basis.

My initial physical therapy treatment targeted pain relief, but I also wanted to make SD contribute to his own treatment by taking part in exercise. It required considerable persuasion to convince SD to begin exercising! I taught him passive extension procedures that involved his lying on the floor and pressing with his arms to encourage restoration of a normal lumbar curve. During this exercise, his pain reduced in intensity, and localized to the lumbar region, shrinking in size. To encourage correct bending, I placed 15-inch-long strips of nonelastic tape on either side of his spine, from the pelvic region to the midthoracic area. As SD bent forward, the tape tightened on the skin, restricting spinal flexion and encouraging him to bend from the knees.

I taught SD pelvic tilting, first passively and then actively, during the first treatment session. Although I instructed him to continue practicing at home, he showed little willingness to do so. I therefore instructed him to visit the company medical center daily, to practice his exercises under supervision of a physical therapy assistant or nurse. He did this each working day for two weeks.

continued

Case History, *continued*

In his second treatment session, I started SD on a single abdominal hollowing exercise, choosing hollowing in wall-supported standing (with a webbing belt) since it was easiest for him to perform. With the use of a mirror, palpation, and surface EMG feedback, he was able to perform consistent hollowing by his third treatment session. I then encouraged him to practice hollowing without aids in wall-support standing, instructing him to draw his abdominal wall away from the waistband of his trousers (without holding his breath) and to hold the contraction for 5-10 seconds. I told him to repeat the exercise 3 times daily for 10 repetitions.

By our third session, the combination of increased flexibility to pelvic tilt and back taping made SD bend more correctly. I assigned hamstring stretching exercises (active knee extension) in a lying position—10 reps, holding each for 10 seconds, during his treatment sessions on alternate working days. I also referred him to the company occupational health nurse for advice on diet and monitored weight loss.

Video feedback helped SD learn correct bending techniques; and he practiced the hip hinge action (with a stick placed along the length of the spine) first with and then without video feedback. After four treatment sessions and 10 days of supervised exercise, SD was pain free. (But I also discovered that SD stopped practicing his exercise program two weeks after treatment began!) I encouraged him to perform the hollowing procedure when walking to his tea break (morning and afternoon) and his lunch break. The action was to contract the muscles to pull away from the waistband, hold the contraction while taking 10 steps, relax for 10 steps, and begin over again— a technique known as "postural walking." I told him to continue this contraction-and-rest procedure for the full length of the walk (about 5 minutes). Because this action was easy to perform and was built into SD's daily activity, he received it well. Three months after his first appointment, SD was still practicing the postural walking procedure daily. He reported a feeling of "strength" in his abdomen, with the added advantage of increased tone and a flatter stomach.

Points to Note

✔ SD had a flatback posture and chronic back pain.

✔ Previous to my seeing him, SD had received only medication and passive physical treatments.

✔ He had taken no active part in the care of his own back condition.

✔ Back taping encouraged him to move more correctly.

✔ Because SD was unwilling to exercise on his own, I arranged for him to do his exercises at work under supervision of a PT assistant.

✔ Although he did not continue abdominal hollowing exercises at home, he liked the "postural walking" approach—which we therefore built into his daily activities.

SUMMARY

- When you first see a client, assess him or her for basic stability, posture, alignment, segmental control, and muscle imbalance.
- Treat pain before proceeding with stability exercises.
- In many cases, your first several sessions will address only the most severe deficiency.
- By the third or fourth session, if not earlier, you generally will want to focus on *all* aspects of stability, prescribing exercises for any area where there is a deficit.
- Prescribe specific exercises for specific goals; there is no such thing as a "general" prescription for back stability.
- The principle of specificity applies also to advanced stability exercises. When prescribing procedures from chapters 8 or 9, target them to your clients' specific goals and needs, whether they are related to the workplace or to the playing field.
- Four case histories provide step-by-step examples of treatment programs for individuals with varying kinds of problems.

11
Preventing Back Injuries and Reinjuries

It is surprising how many people go to a great deal of effort to follow a rehabilitation program after a back injury, only to reinjure the back by doing something foolish at home or at work. I strongly urge you to take a few minutes to go over the information in this chapter with your clients so that they will have an increased probability of maintaining the progress you've helped them achieve.

In the large majority of cases, according to my experience, you will meet with mild resistance or even boredom, because most people will say (at least to themselves if not to you), "Yes, yes, I know all that, use your legs and not your back, don't bend over. . . ." Yet a significant number of these same people will end up doing something outrageously silly because they haven't internalized proper safety procedures. I suggest that you actually role play these ideas with your clients. After leading them through the information in this chapter, take just 5 or 10 minutes to point to various objects and say, "All right, let's say you have to carry that chair into the next room and set it against the wall. Plan it out for me, explain to me the proper lifting/carrying procedure, then show me how you would position yourself for the lift." (I *don't* suggest letting anyone do a heavy or awkward lift, for reasons of liability.)

KEEP THE SPINE VERTICAL

Merely reaching over a table can tremendously leverage the stress on the spine. Picking up a mug of coffee from the opposite side of a table, for example, can produce more force against the intervertebral disks than lifting a 20-pound weight next to one's body. Remember, torque = force × the length of the lever arm. If the spine remains vertical, leverage is minimal. If the spine is allowed to move toward the horizontal, higher leverage forces increase the tendency for the spine to flex, loading the spinal tissues. An analogy: when a flexible fishing rod is held vertically, it remains straight; if you tilt it, it bends under its own weight. In order to keep the rod straight in a tilted or horizontal position, you must support its weight. The same principle applies to the back. If you want to move your back away from the vertical, you should support it by placing your hand onto a nearby tabletop or chair or whatever, or onto your knee if nothing else is available. The additional support greatly reduces the stress on the spine and enables you to maintain correct alignment.

Repeated flexion also adds to spinal stress, greatly increasing discal pressure and continually stretching the posterior spinal tissues. Ov r time, repeated flexion can lead to tissue breakdown. Microtrauma of this type gives rise to classical postural pain syndromes (McKenzie 1981). Instruct your clients to reduce their total amount of bending in any one day by using more effective movements and by improving general back care. Figure 11.1 shows examples of poor general back care, along with alternatives for reducing stress on the spine.

KEY POINT: Support the spine whenever it is not vertical, and reduce the total amount of bending.

PRINCIPLES OF LIFTING IN THE HOME AND ON THE JOB

Both at home and at work, your clients should follow the principles of good back stability in any lifting or other manual tasks. Most simply stated, they must *plan* their actions carefully and *minimize* the forces of the lift.

Planning

Planning prevents surprises. One of the most common reasons for lifting injuries is failure to assess the entire situation before trying to move an object. Tell your clients they must evaluate three areas:

1. **Assess the environment.** Note the floor surface. Is it uneven? Is it wet? Are there potential trip hazards? They should plan the entire path over which they will carry the object. Does the path involve going through a doorway? If so, is it accessible and open? Is it wide enough? (It is amazing how often people will carry a couch or desk up to a doorway, only to discover the opening is too small!) Where is the object to be placed? If it is to go on a table, is there room for it or do other items need to be moved first?

2. **Assess the object.** The distribution of the object's weight can be even more important than the absolute weight. The heaviest part of the object should be held close to the body to reduce the leverage effect, and

Correct ✓   **Incorrect** ✗

Vacuuming

Removing clothes
from the dryer

Reaching for object
on a high shelf

Lifting (or even
talking with)
a small child

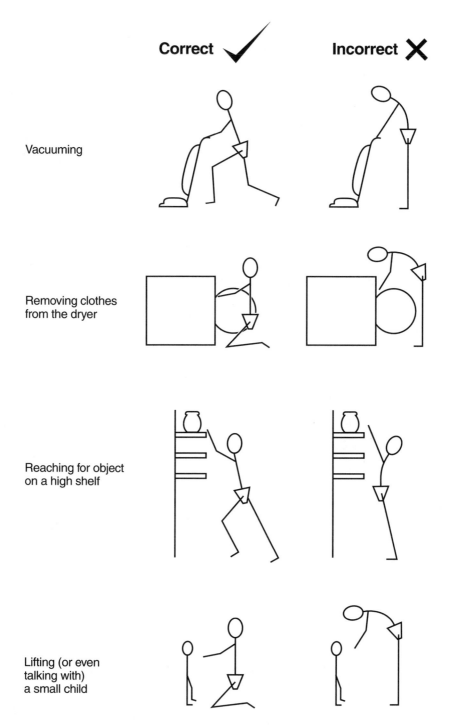

Figure 11.1 Proper and improper back care in the home.

individuals must feel comfortable with the weight lifted in relation to their own health status, training, and capability. They should consider the size *and* shape of the object: a light object that is very bulky or that may shift (e.g., a container of powder or fluid) offers a greater potential for injury. They must also consider any possible danger from the contents—if a container holds acid, or a scalding liquid, what would happen in the event of an unforeseen accident?

3. **Assess themselves.** Do they feel confident that a lift is within their capability? Individuals with a knee injury, for example, may not be able to bend their knees sufficiently to lift the object in a correct manner. Are there any relevant medical conditions? Pregnant women should severely restrict their lifting; and individuals with heart disease, low back pain, or hip pathology will have reduced capacities. Many people injure their backs by trying to lift objects they suspected were too heavy for them. I often hear something like "I was afraid I couldn't lift it, but it had to be moved and I didn't have time to find help" when I examine people following back injuries. Especially in men, "machismo" is a very common and very dangerous attitude. Emphasize to your clients that it is in no way "wimpy" to admit they should not lift a given item. Such a statement in fact shows great wisdom and maturity. If special training is generally needed before a certain kind of lift, and if a person has not received that training, he certainly must not attempt it. In general, *if individuals are unsure about any aspect of a lift, they should not attempt it.*

> **KEY POINT:** Individuals should not attempt *any* lift if they have the slightest doubts about their abilities to perform the lift safely.

Minimizing the Stress of a Lift

There are several ways to reduce the physical stress of a lift.

The Safe Zone

The center of gravity of the human body typically lies at the S2/S3 level. Pulling an object near to this "safe zone" reduces the leverage forces acting on the body; allowing the object to move farther away from this point increases the leverage and therefore the stress. If holding an object within the safe zone next to the pelvis represents 100% lifting capacity, this capacity is reduced by 20% when the object is held a forearm's length from the body, and by 75% when the object is lifted at arm's length.

Teach your clients to pull objects they are lifting toward the body's center of gravity at the sacrum—to pull them into the safe zone *as soon as* possible and keep them there *as long as* possible. When lifting something from the floor, they should pull it in toward the body early in the lift by sliding the object along the floor. Only when the object is pulled close to the safe zone should the lift begin. Although it may not be possible to keep the object within the safe zone during the entire lift, the longer it is held there, the better. If a lift takes a total of 15 seconds to complete, it will be performed far more safely if the object is within the safe zone for 12 of the 15 seconds than if it is there for only 5 seconds. Since the lift takes the same total time in each case, lifting safely will not slow a person down.

KEY POINT: Pull an object into the "safe zone" (near the sacrum) as soon as possible during a lift, and keep it there for as long as possible.

Appropriate Stance and Grip

Instruct your clients to use **two hands** when lifting a heavy object from the floor. They should stand at the corner of the object, with the feet at 90° to each other (figure 11.2). With this foot position, the knees pass to the

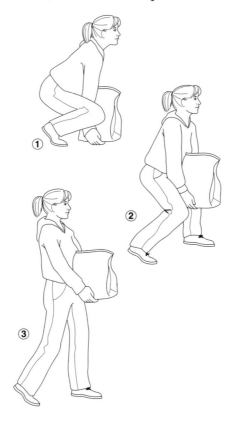

Figure 11.2 Double-handed lift.

sides of the object as they are bent. At least one foot must stay flat on the floor, to aid stability.

The hands should grip under the object ("hook grip") rather than merely at its sides, to avoid their slipping—elbows in to aid power; knees bent; the back aligned and near vertical for the majority of the lift (only when the object is approaching the floor, when the individual is setting it down, is the back allowed to flex slightly). Individuals should look up as they lift, to aid the general feeling of back extension; and their hips should remain below the shoulders at all times.

For certain heavy, large objects such as a sack of grain or a bag of concrete (figure 11.3), suggest a modification of the double-handed lift called

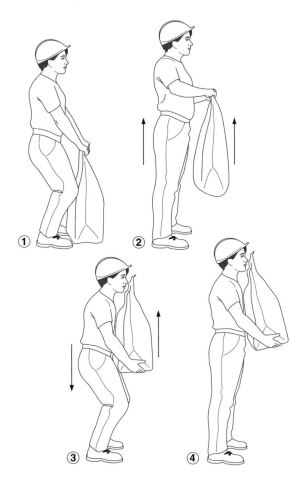

Figure 11.3 (1) Bend knees to get close to the sack, gripping it at the top; (2) rapidly straighten the legs and pull the sack up high; (3) dip down beneath the sack as its momentum continues to carry it upward; (4) straighten the legs to stand up, holding the sack high against the chest.

a snatch lift. The **snatch lift** uses speed and momentum to reduce the strength needed for the lift, but is only possible for objects that can be grasped at the top. It is highly effective, but requires great skill and therefore practice. Since it is performed rapidly, there is little margin for error. The person lifting uses a position similar to that used for the double-handed lift, except the squat is not as deep. Gripping the object *at its top*, the individual keeps his back straight and his legs somewhat bent. The action is to rapidly straighten the legs and raise onto the toes (as with the power clean exercise, page 221) while pulling the object upward. Most of the power for the lift comes from the legs, the arm pull being used mostly to transmit the power and guide the path of the object. The object's momentum carries it upward—and at the height of its movement (when its weight feels minimal), the individual changes his grip to place his hands under the object and pull it firmly into the safe zone.

Single-handed lifts are appropriate for lighter objects (figure 11.4). The individual should assume a lunge position, with feet shoulder-width apart and one foot forward of the other. If the right hand is used to lift, the left foot leads the movement and the left hand may be placed on the left knee for support. The back remains in its neutral position and is kept near the vertical throughout the lift. The knee of the forward leg should pass just over the foot, but no farther, so that the tibia of the leading leg is nearly vertical—this way the individual will be pressing her hand down on a more stable lower leg. If the leading foot is dorsiflexed too far, the hand pressing down on the knee will increase the range of dorsiflexion and make it more difficult to raise the body from the ground.

Pushing and pulling activities can also place considerable stress on the back if they are performed incorrectly. It is essential that back alignment is maintained, and that the power for the movement comes from the legs rather than from the spine. Instruct your clients to begin a push either facing forward with their hands on the object and their arms straight, or facing backward with their backs flat against the object. In either case, they should keep their pelvises in neutral position and produce most of the power for pushing/pulling in the legs—power that is directed through the straight, stable spine to the object being moved. Make sure your clients know to take only small steps during the push/pull—overly large steps will overstretch the body and pull the spine out of alignment.

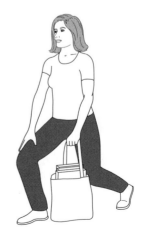

Figure 11.4 Single-handed lift.

SUMMARY

- Individuals should keep their spines vertical, or as near vertical as possible, during a lift.
- Repeated spinal flexion during lifting can lead to serious breakdown of tissues.
- Whenever the spine is not vertical, it should be supported by placing a hand either on a stable object or on the bent knee.
- Before lifting any object, individuals should plan the move: they should assess the environment, the object, and their own capabilities.
- If there is *any* doubt in individuals' minds that they can safely lift/ carry an object, they should refrain from doing so.
- The "safe zone" is near the sacrum, since the average person's center of gravity is at approximately the S2/S3 level. Lifted objects should be brought to the safe zone as quickly as possible, and remain there as long as possible.
- Individuals should use two hands to lift heavy objects. When lifting lighter objects with only one hand, they should place the free hand on a bent knee to provide support for the spine.
- The "snatch lift" is useful for lifting heavy objects that can be grasped at the top, but the movement is difficult and should be practiced before it is used.

Bibliography

Adams, M. 1989. Letter to the editor. *Spine* 14:1272.

Adams, M.A., and Dolan, P. 1997. The combined function of the spine, pelvis, and legs when lifting with a straight back. In *Movement, stability and low back pain*, ed. A. Vleeming, V. Mooney, T. Dorman, C. Snijders, and R. Stoeckart. New York: Churchill Livingstone.

Adams, M.A., and Hutton, W.C. 1983. The mechanical function of the lumbar apophyseal joints *Spine* 8:327-30.

Adams, M.A.; Hutton, W.C.; and Stott, J.R.R. 1980. The resistance to flexion of the lumbar intervertebral joint. *Spine* 5:245-53.

Adams, M.A.; McNally, D.S.; Chinn, H.; and Dolan, P. 1994. Posture and the compressive strength of the lumbar spine. *Clinical Biomechanics* 9:5-14.

Allan, D.B., and Waddell, G. 1989. An historical perspective on low back pain and disability. *Acta Orthop Scand* (Suppl) 60:1-5.

Allison, G.; Kendle, K.; Roll, S.; Schupelius, J.; Scott, Q.; and Panizza, J. 1998. The role of the diaphragm during abdominal hollowing exercises. *Australian Journal of Physiotherapy* 44:95-102.

Andersson, E.; Oddsson, L.; Grundstrom, H.; and Thorstensson, A. 1995. The role of the psoas and iliacus muscles for stability and movement of the lumbar spine, pelvis and hip. *Scandinavian Journal of Medicine and Science in Sports* 5:10-16.

Appell, H.J. 1990. Muscular atrophy following immobilisation: a review. *Sports Medicine* 10:42-58.

Aruin, A.S., and Latach, M.L. 1995. Directional specificity of postural muscles in feed-forward postural reactions during fast voluntary arm movements. *Experimental Brain Research* 103:323-32.

Aspden, R.M. 1987. Intra-abdominal pressure and its role in spinal mechanics. *Clinical Biomechanics* 2:168-74.

Aspden, R.M. 1989. The spine as an arch. A new mathematical model. *Spine* 14:266-74.

Aspden, R.M. 1992. Review of the functional anatomy of the spinal ligaments and the lumbar erector spinae muscles. *Clinical Anatomy* 5:372-87.

Atkinson, H.W. 1986. Principles of treatment. In *Cash's textbook of neurology for physiotherapists*, 4th edition, ed. P.A Downie. London: Faber and Faber.

Baechle, T.R. 1994. *Essentials of strength training and conditioning*. Champaign, IL: Human Kinetics.

Bandy, W.D., and Irion, J.M. 1994. The effect of time on static stretch of the flexibility of the hamstring muscles. *Physical Therapy* 74:845-52.

Barrack, R.L., and Skinner, H.B. 1990. The sensory function of knee ligaments. In *Knee ligaments: structure, function, and injury*, ed. D. Daniel. New York: Raven Press.

Barrack, R.L.; Skinner, H.B.; and Brunet, G. 1983. Joint kinesthesia in the highly trained knee. *Journal of Sports Medicine and Physical Fitness* 24:18-20.

Barrett, D.S.; Cobb, A.G.; and Bentley, G. 1991. Joint proprioception in normal, osteoarthritic, and replaced knees. *Journal of Bone and Joint Surgery* 73B:53-56.

Bartelink, D.L. 1957. The role of abdominal pressure in relieving the pressure on the lumbar intervertebral discs. *Journal of Bone and Joint Surgery* 39B:718-25.

Bastide, G.; Zadeh, J.; and Lefebre, D. 1989. Are the little muscles what we think they are? *Surgical and Radiological Anatomy* 11:255-56.

Beard, D.J.; Kyberd, P.J.; O'Connor, J.J.; Fergusson, C.M.; and Dodd, C.A.F. 1994. Reflex hamstring contraction latency in anterior cruciate ligament deficiency. *Journal of Orthopaedic Research* 12:219-28.

Beiring-Sorensen, R. 1984. Physical measurement as risk indicators for low back trouble over a one year period. *Spine* 9:106-19.

Bernhardt, M.; White, A.A.; Panjabi, M.M. 1992. Lumbar spine instability. In *The lumbar spine and back pain*. 4th ed., ed. M.I.V. Jayson. Edinburgh: Churchill Livingstone.

Bernier, J.N., and Perrin, D.H. 1998. Effect of coordination training on proprioception of the functionally unstable ankle. *Journal of Orthopedic and Sports Physical Therapy* 27:264-75.

Biedermann, H.J.; Shanks, G.L.; Forrest, W.J.; and Inglis, J. 1991. Power spectrum analyses of electromyographic activity. *Spine* 16:1179-84.

Boden, S.D.; Davis, D.O.; and Dina, T.S. 1990. Abnormal magnetic resonance scans of the lumbar spine in asymptomatic subjects. *Journal of Bone and Joint Surgery* [Am] 72:403.

Bogduk, N.; and Engel, R. 1984. The menisci of the lumbar zygapophyseal joints. A review of their anatomy and clinical significance. *Spine* 9:454-60.

Bogduk, N.; and Jull, G. 1985. The theoretical pathology of acute locked back: a basis for manipulative therapy. *Manual Medicine* 1:78-82.

Bogduk, N.; Pearcy, M.; and Hadfield, G. 1992. Anatomy and biomechanics of psoas major. *Clinical Biomechanics* 7:109-19.

Bogduk, N., and Twomey, L.T. 1987. *Clinical anatomy of the lumbar spine.* Edinburgh: Churchill Livingstone.

Bogduk, N., and Twomey, L.T. 1991. *Clinical anatomy of the lumbar spine.* 2d ed. Edinburgh: Churchill Livingstone.

Bradford, F.K., and Spurling, R.G. 1945. *The intervertebral disc.* Springfield, IL: Charles C. Thomas.

Bullock-Saxton, J. 1988. Normal and abnormal postures in the sagittal plane and their relationship to low back pain. *Physiotherapy Practice* 4:94-104.

Bullock-Saxton, J. 1993. Postural alignment in standing: a repeatability study. *Australian Journal of Physiotherapy* 39:25-29.

Bullock-Saxton, J.E.; Bullock, M.I.; Tod, C.; Riley, D.R.; and Morgan, A.E. 1991. Postural stability in young adult men and women. *New Zealand Journal of Physiotherapy* 3:7-10.

Bush, K.; Cowan, N.; and Katz, D.E. 1992. The natural history of sciatica associated with disc pathology: a prospective study with clinical and independent radiographic follow up. *Spine* 17:1205-12.

Cailliet, R. 1981. *Low back pain syndrome.* 3d ed. Philadelphia: Davis.

Cailliet, R. 1983. *Soft tissue pain and disability.* Philadelphia: Davis.

Chartered Society of Physiotherapy (CSP). 1998. *Low back pain. Information for sufferers.* [Online]. Available: **http://www.csp.org.uk** [October 15, 1999].

Cappozzo, A.; Felici, F.; Figura, F.; and Gazzani, F. 1985. Lumbar spine loading during half-squat exercises. *Medicine and Science in Sports and Exercise* 17(5):613-20.

Cholewicki, J., and McGill, S.M. 1992. Lumbar posterior ligament involvement during extremely heavy lifts estimated from fluoroscopic measurements. *Journal of Biomechanics* 25(1):17-28.

Comerford, M. 1995. Muscle imbalance. Course notes. Nottingham School of Physiotherapy.

Comerford, M. 1998. Dynamic stability. Physiotools compatible computer programme. Physiotools development office. Pihapolku F. 02420. Jorvas. Finland.

Cornwall, M.W.; Melinda, P.B.; and Barry, S. 1991. Effect of mental practice on isometric muscular strength. *Journal of Orthopedic and Sports Physical Therapy* 13:217-23.

Cresswell, A.G.; Grundstrom, H.; and Thorstensson, A. 1992. Observations on intra-abdominal pressure and patterns of abdominal intra-muscular activity in man. *Acta Physiol Scand* 144:409-18.

Cresswell, A.G.; Oddsson, L.; and Thorstensson, A. 1994. The influence of sudden perturbations on trunk muscle activity and intra-abdominal pressure while standing. *Experimental Brain Research* 98:336-41.

Crock, H.V., and Yoshizawa, H. 1976. The blood supply of the lumbar vertebral column. *Clinical Orthopaedics* 115:6-21.

Crowell, R.D.; Cummings, G.S.; Walker, J.R.; and Tillman, L.J. 1994. Intratester and intertester reliability and validity of measures on innominate bone inclination. *Journal of Orthopedic and Sports Physical Therapy* 20:88-97.

Davis, P.R., and Troup, J.D.G. 1964. Pressures in the trunk cavities when pulling, pushing, and lifting. *Ergonomics* 7:465-74.

Day, J.W.; Smidt, G.L.; and Lehmann, T. 1984. Effect of pelvic tilt on standing posture. *Physical Therapy* 64:510-16.

Delitto, R.S.; Rose, S.J.; and Apts, D.W. 1987. Electromyographic analysis of two techniques for squat lifting. *Physical Therapy* 67:1329-34.

Deutsch, F.E. 1996. Isolated lumbar strengthening in the rehabilitation of chronic low back pain. *Journal of Manipulative and Physiological Therapeutics* 19:124-33.

Deyo, R.A.; Diehl, A.K.; and Rosenthal, M. 1986. How many days of bed rest for acute low back pain. *New England Journal of Medicine* 315:1064.

Eie, N. 1966. Load capacity of the low back. *Journal of Oslo City Hospitals* 16:73-98.

Enoka, R.M. 1988. *Neuromechanical basis of kinesiology.* Champaign, IL: Human Kinetics.

Etnyre, B.R., and Abraham, L.D. 1986. H-reflex changes during static stretching and two variations of proprioceptive neuromuscular facilitation techniques. *Electroencephalography and Clinical Neurophysiology* 63:174-79.

Etnyre, B.R., and Lee, E.J. 1987. Comments on proprioceptive neuromuscular facilitation stretching. *Research Quarterly for Exercise and Sport* 58:184-88.

Fansler, C.L.; Poff, C.L.; and Shepard, K.F. 1985. Effects of mental practice on balance in elderly women. *Physical Therapy* 65:1332-38.

Farfan, H.F. 1988. Biomechanics of the lumbar spine. In *Managing low back pain.* 2d ed., ed. W.H. Kirkaldy-Willis. London: Churchill Livingstone.

Farfan, H.F.; Osteria, V.; and Lamy, C. 1976. The mechanical etiology of spondylolysis and spondylolisthesis. *Clinical Orthopedics and Related Research* 117:40-55.

Freeman, M.A.R.; Dean, M.R.E.; and Hanham, I.W.F. 1965. The etiology and prevention of functional instability of the foot. *Journal of Bone and Joint Surgery* 47B(4):678-85.

Friedli, W.G.; Hallet, M.; and Simon, S.R. 1984. Postural adjustments associated with rapid voluntary arm movements. Electromyographic data. *Journal of Neurology, Neurosurgery and Psychiatry* 47:611-22.

Frymoyer, J.W., and Cats-Baril, W.L. 1991. An overview of the incidences and costs of low back pain. *Orthopedic Clinics of North America* 22:263.

Frymoyer, J.W., and Gordon, S.L. 1989. *Symposium on new perspectives on low back pain.* Park Ridge, IL: American Academy of Orthopedic Surgeons.

Goldspink, G. 1992. Cellular and molecular aspects of adaptation in skeletal muscle. In *Strength and power in sport*, ed. P.V. Komi. Oxford: Blackwell.

Goldspink, G. 1996. Personal communication.

Gossman, M.R.; Sahrmann, S.A.; and Rose, S.J. 1982. Review of length associated changes in muscle. *Physical Therapy* 62:1799-808.

Gracovetsky, S.; Farfan, H.F.; and Helleur, C. 1985. The abdominal mechanism. *Spine* 10:317-24.

Gracovetsky, S.; Kary, M.; Levy, S.; Ben Said, R.; Pitchen, I.; and Helie, J. 1990. Analysis of spinal and muscular activity during flexion/extension and free lifts. *Spine* 15:1333-39.

Gracovetsky, S.; Farfan, H.F.; and Lamy, C. 1977. A mathematical model of the lumbar spine using an optimal system to control muscles and ligaments. *Orthopaedic Clinics of North America* 8:135-53.

Guimaraes, A.C.S.; Vaz, M.A.; De Campos, M.I.A.; and Marantes, R. 1991. The contribution of the rectus abdominis and rectus femoris in twelve selected abdominal exercises. *Journal of Sports Medicine and Physical Fitness* 31:222-30.

Harman E.; Frykman, P.; Clagett, B.; and Kraemer, W. 1988. Intra-abdominal and intra-thoracic pressures during lifting and jumping. *Medicine and Science in Sports and Exercise* 20:195-201.

Hart, D.L, and Rose, S.J. 1986. Reliability of a non-invasive method for measuring the lumbar curve. *Journal of Orthopedic and Sports Physical Therapy* 8:180-84.

Hemborg, B.; Moritz, U.; and Hamberg, J. 1983. Intra-abdominal pressure and trunk muscle activity during lifting—effect of abdominal muscle training in healthy subjects. *Scandinavian Journal of Rehabilitation Medicine* 15:183-96.

Hemborg B.; Moritz, U.; Hamberg, J.; Holmstrom, E.; Lowing, H.; and Akesson, I. 1985. Intra-abdominal pressure and trunk muscle activity during lifting. III. Effects of abdominal muscle training in chronic low-back patients. *Scandinavian Journal of Rehabilitation Medicine* 17:15-24.

Hides, J.A.; Richardson, C.A.; and Jull, G.A. 1996. Multifidus muscle recovery is not automatic after resolution of acute, first-episode low back pain. *Spine* 21:2763-69.

Hides, J.A.; Stokes, M.J.; Saide, M.; Jull, G.A.; and Cooper, D.H. 1994. Evidence of lumbar multifidus muscle wasting ipsilateral to symptoms in patients with acute/subacute low back pain. *Spine* 19: 165-72.

Hirsch, C. and Schajowicz, F. 1952. Studies on structural changes in the lumbar annulus fibrosis. *Acta Orthopaedica Scandinavica* 22:184-89.

Hirsch, C., and Nachemson, A. 1954. New observations on mechanical behaviour of lumbar discs. *Acta Orthopaedica Scandinavica* 23:254-83.

Hodges, P.W., and Richardson, C.A. 1996. Contraction of transversus abdominis invariably precedes movement of the upper and lower limb. In *Proceedings of the 6th International Conference of the International Federation of Orthopaedic Manipulative Therapists.* Lillehammer, Norway.

Hodges, P.; Richardson, C.; and Jull, G. 1996. Evaluation of the relationship between laboratory and clinical tests of transversus abdominis function. *Physiotherapy Research International* 1:30-40.

Holm, S.; Maroudas, A.; Urban, J.P.G.; Selstam, G.; and Nachemson, A. 1981. Nutrition of the intervertebral disc: solute transport and metabolism. *Connect Tissue Res* 8:101-19.

Holt, L.E., and Smith, R. 1983. *The effect of selected stretching programs on active and passive flexibility.* Del Mar, CA: Research Center for Sport.

Hughes, M.A.; Duncan, P.W.; Rose, D.K.; Chandler, J.M.; and Studenski, S.A. 1996. The relationship of postural sway to sensorimotor function, functional performance, and disability in the elderly. *Archives of Physical Medicine and Rehabilitation* 77:567-72.

Hukins, D.W.L. 1987. Properties of spinal materials. In *The lumbar spine and back pain,* ed. M.I.V. Jayson. Edinburgh: Churchill Livingstone.

Hukins, D.W.L.; Aspden, R.M.; and Hickey, D.S. 1990. Thoracolumbar fascia can increase the efficiency of the erector spinae muscles. *Clinical Biomechanics* 5:30-34.

Hyman, J., and Liebenson, C. 1996. Spinal stabilization exercise program. In *Rehabilitation of the spine,* ed. C. Liebenson. Baltimore: Williams & Wilkins.

Irion, J.M. 1992. Use of the gym ball in rehabilitation of spinal dysfunction. In *Orthopaedic physical therapy clinics of North America.* Oxford: Churchill Livingstone.

Jacob, H.A.C., and Kissling, R.O. 1995. The mobility of the sacroiliac joints in healthy volunteers between 20 and 50 years of age. *Clinical Biomechanics* 10:352-61.

Janda, V. 1986. Muscle weakness and inhibition pseudoparesis in back pain syndromes. In *Modern manual therapy,* ed. G. Grieve. Edinburgh: Churchill Livingstone.

Janda, V. 1992. Muscle imbalance and musculoskeletal pain. Course notes. University of Oxford. UK.

Janda, V. 1993. Muscle strength in relation to muscle length, pain and muscle imbalance. In *Muscle strength. International perspectives in physical therapy,* ed. K. Harms-Ringdahl. Edinburgh: Churchill Livingstone.

Janda V., and Schmid, H.J.A. 1980. Muscles as a pathogenic factor in back pain. *Proceedings of the International Federation of Orthopaedic Manipulative Therapists, 4th Conference,* 17-18. New Zealand.

Jensel, M.C.; Brant-Zawadzki, M.N.; and Obuchowki, N. 1994. Magnetic resonance imaging of the lumbar spine in people without back pain. *New England Journal of Medicine* 2:69.

Johnson, C., and Reid, J.G. 1991. Lumbar compressive and shear forces during various curl up exercises. *Clinical Biomechanics* 6:97-104.

Jorgensen, K., and Nicolaisen, T. 1987. Trunk extensor endurance: determination and relation to low-back trouble. *Ergonomics* 30:259-67.

Jull, G.A. 1994. Headaches of cervical origin. In *Physical therapy of the cervical and thoracic spine,* ed. R. Grant. New York: Churchill Livingstone.

Jull, G.A., and Janda, V. 1987. Muscles and motor control in low back pain: assessment and management. In *Physical therapy of the low back,* ed. L.T. Twomey. New York: Churchill Livingstone.

Jull, G., and Richardson, C.A. 1994a. Active stabilisation of the trunk. Course notes. University of Edinburgh.

Jull, G.A., and Richardson, C.A. 1994b. Rehabilitation of active stabilization of the lumbar spine. In *Physical therapy of the low back.* 2d ed., ed. L.T. Twomey and L.T. Taylor. Edinburgh: Churchill Livingstone.

Kapandji, I. 1974. *The physiology of joints, vol. 3. The spine.* London: Churchill Livingstone.

Kendall, F.P.; McCreary, E.K.; and Provance, P.G. 1993. *Muscles. Testing and function.* 4th ed. Baltimore: Williams & Wilkins.

Kennedy, J.C.; Alexander, I.J.; and Hayes, K.C. 1982. Nerve supply of the human knee and its functional importance. *American Journal of Sports Medicine* 10:329.

Kent, M. 1994. *The Oxford dictionary of sports science and medicine.* Oxford: Oxford University Press.

Kesson, M., and Atkins, E. 1998. *Orthopaedic medicine. A practical approach.* Oxford: Butterworth Heinemann.

Kippers, V., and Parker, A.W. 1984. Posture related to myoelectric silence of erectores spinae during trunk flexion. *Spine* 9:740-45.

Kirby, M.C.; Sikoryn, T.A.; Hukins, D.W.L.; and Aspden, R.M. 1989. Structure and mechanical properties of the longitudinal ligaments and ligamentum flavum of the spine. *Journal of Biomedical Engineering* 11:192-96.

Kirkaldy-Willis, W.H. 1990. *The lumbar spine.* New York: Saunders.

Klein, J.A., and Hukins, D.W.L. 1983. Relocation of the bending axis during flexion-extension of the lumbar intervertebral discs and its implications for prolapse. *Spine* 8: 659-64.

Koh, T.J. 1995. Do adaptations in serial sarcomere number occur with strength training? *Human Movement Science* 14:61-77.

Konradsen, L., and Ravn, J.B. 1990. Ankle instability cause by prolonged peroneal reaction time. *Acta Orthop Scand* 61:388-90.

Kraemer, J.; Kolditz, D.; and Gowin, R. 1985. Water and electrolyte content of human intervertebral discs under variable load. *Spine* 10:69-71.

Lacote, M.; Chevalier, A.M.; Miranda, A.; Bleton, J.P.; and Stevenin, P. 1987. *Clinical evaluation of muscle function.* Edinburgh: Churchill Livingstone.

Lavignolle, B.; Vital, J.M.; and Senegas, J. 1983. An approach to the functional anatomy of the sacroiliac joints in vivo. *Anatomia Clinica* 5:169-76.

Leatt, P.; Reilly, T.; and Troup, J.G.D. 1986. Spinal loading during circuit weight-training and running. *British Journal of Sports Medicine* 20(3):119-24.

Lee, D.G. 1994. Kinematics of the pelvic joints. In *Grieve's modern manual therapy,* ed. J.D. Boyling and N. Palastanga. Edinburgh: Churchill Livingstone.

Lentell, G.L.; Katzman, L.L.; and Walters, M.R. 1990. The relationship between muscle function and ankle stability. *Journal of Orthopedic and Sports Physical Therapy* 11:605-11.

Lephart, S.M., and Fu, F.H. 1995. The role of proprioception in the treatment of sports injuries. *Sports Exercise and Injury* 1:96-102.

Lephart, S.M.; Warner, J.P.; Borsa, P.A.; and Fu, F.H. 1994. Proprioception of the shoulder in normal, unstable, and surgical individuals. *Journal of Shoulder and Elbow Surgery* 3:224-28.

Lester, M.N., and Posner-Mayer, J. 1993. *Spinal stabilisation: utilizing the Swiss ball video.* Denver: Ball Dynamics.

Levine, D.; Walker, J.R.; and Tillman, L.J. 1997. The effect of abdominal muscle strengthening on pelvic tilt and lumbar lordosis. *Physiotherapy Theory and Practice* 13:217-26.

Lewit, K. 1991. *Manipulative therapy in rehabilitation of the locomotor system.* 2d ed. Oxford: Butterworth Heinemann.

Liebenson, C. 1996. *Rehabilitation of the spine.* Baltimore: Williams & Wilkins.

Lieber, R.L. 1992. *Skeletal muscle structure and function.* Baltimore: Williams & Wilkins.

Linsenbardt, S.T.; Thomas, T.R.; and Madsen, R.W. 1992. Effect of breathing techniques on blood pressure response to resistance exercise. *British Journal of Sports Medicine* 26:97-100.

Lipetz, S., and Gutin, B. 1970. An electromyographic study of four abdominal exercises. *Medicine and Science in Sports and Exercise* 2:35-38.

Long, D.M. 1995. Effectiveness of therapies currently employed for persistent low back and leg pain. *Pain Forum* 4:122-25.

Lord, S.R.; Ward, J.A.; Williams, P.; and Zivanovic, E. 1996. The effects of a community exercise program on fracture risk factors in older women. *Osteoporosis International* 6:361-67.

Lovell, F.W.; Rothstein, J.M.; and Personius, W.J. 1989. Reliability of clinical measurements of lumbar lordosis taken with a flexible rule. *Physical Therapy* 69:96-105.

Luttgens, K.; and Wells, K. 1982. *Kinesiology. Scientific basis and human motion.* 7th ed. Philadelphia: Saunders College Publishing.

Macintosh, J.E., and Bogduk, N. 1986. The biomechanics of the lumbar multifidus. *Clinical Biomechanics* 1:205-13.

Macintosh, J.E., and Bogduk, N. 1987. The anatomy and function of the lumbar back muscles and their fascia. In *Physical therapy of the low back,* ed. L.T. Twomey. New York: Churchill Livingstone.

Macintosh, J.E.; Bogduk, N.; and Gracovetsky, S. 1987. The biomechanics of the thoracolumbar fascia. *Clinical Biomechanics* 2:78-83.

Main, C.J., and Watson, P.J. 1996. Guarded movements: development of chronicity. *Journal of Musculoskeletal Pain* 4:163-70.

Maitland, G.D. 1986. *Vertebral manipulation.* 5th ed. London: Butterworths.

Markolf, K.L., and Morris, J.M. 1974. The structural components of the intervertebral disc. *Journal of Bone and Joint Surgery* 56A:675-87.

McConnell, J. 1993. Promoting effective segmental alignment. In *Key issues in musculoskeletal physiotherapy,* ed. J. Crosbie and J. McConnell. Oxford: Butterworth Heinemann.

McGill, S.M. 1997. Distribution of tissue loads in the low back during a variety of daily and rehabilitation tasks. *Journal of Rehabilitation Research and Development* 34:448-58.

McGill, S.M. 1998. Low back exercises: evidence for improving exercise regimens. *Physical Therapy* 78:754-65.

McGill, S.M., and Norman, R.W. 1986. Partitioning of the L4-L5 dynamic moment into disc, ligamentous, and muscular components during lifting. *Spine* 11:666-78.

McGill, S.M.; Norman, R.W.; and Sharratt, M.T. 1990. The effect of an abdominal belt on trunk muscles activity and intra-abdominal pressure during squat lifts. *Ergonomics* 33:147-60.

McGill, S.M.; Juker, D.; and Kropf, P. 1996. Quantitative intramuscular myoelectric activity of quadratus lumborum during a wide variety of tasks. *Clinical Biomechanics* 11:170-72.

McKenzie, R.A. 1981. *The lumbar spine. Mechanical diagnosis and therapy.* Lower Hutt, New Zealand: Spinal Publications.

McKenzie, R.A. 1990. *The cervical and thoracic spine. Mechanical diagnosis and therapy.* Lower Hutt, New Zealand: Spinal Publications.

Miller, J.A.A.; Haderspeck, K.A.; and Schultz, A.B. 1983. Posterior element loads in lumbar motion segments. *Spine* 8:331-37.

Miller, M.I., and Medeiros, J.M. 1987. Recruitment of internal oblique and transversus abdominis muscles during the eccentric phase of the curl-up exercise. *Physical Therapy* 67:1213-17.

Moore, M.A., and Kukulka, C.G. 1991. Depression of Hoffman reflexes following voluntary contraction and implications for proprioceptive neuromuscular facilitation therapy. *Physical Therapy* 71:321-33.

Morgan, D.L., and Lynn, R. 1994. Decline running produces more sarcomeres in rat vastus intermedius muscle fibers than does incline running. *Journal of Applied Physiology* 77:1439-44.

Morris, J.M.; Lucas, D.B.; and Bresler, B. 1961. Role of the trunk in stability of the spine. *Journal of Bone and Joint Surgery (Am)* 43A:327-51.

Mottram, S.L. 1997. Dynamic stability of the scapula. *Manual Therapy* 2:123-31.

Murray, M.P.; Seireg, A.; and Sepic, S.B. 1975. Normal postural stability and steadiness: quantitative assessment. *Journal of Bone and Joint Surgery* 57A:510-16.

Nachemson, A.L. 1992. Newest knowledge of low back pain. *Clinical Orthopaedics* 279:8.

Nachemson, A., and Evans, J. 1968. Some mechanical properties of the third lumbar laminar ligament (ligamentum flavum). *Journal of Biomechanics* 1:211.

Ng, G., and Richardson, C.A. 1990. The effects of training triceps surae using progressive speed loading. *Physiotherapy Practice* 6:77-84.

Ng, G., and Richardson, C. 1994. EMG study of erector spinae and multifidus in two isometric back extension exercises. *Australian Journal of Physiotherapy* 40:115-21.

Norkin, C.C., and Levangie, P.K. 1992. *Joint structure and function. A comprehensive analysis.* 2d ed. Philadelphia: Davis.

Norris, C.M. 1993. Abdominal muscle training in sport. *British Journal of Sports Medicine* 27:19-27.

Norris, C.M. 1994b. Abdominal training. Dangers and exercise modifications. *Physiotherapy in Sport* 14:10-14.

Norris, C.M. 1994c. Taping: components, applications and mechanisms. *Sports Exercise and Injury* 1:14-17.

Norris, C.M. 1995a. Spinal stabilisation 2. Limiting factors to end-range motion in the lumbar spine. *Physiotherapy* 81:4-12.

Norris, C.M. 1995b. *Weight training. Principles and practice.* London: A&C Black.

Norris, C.M. 1997. *Abdominal training.* London: A&C Black.

Norris, C.M. 1998. *Sports Injuries. Diagnosis and management.* 2d ed. Oxford: Butterworth Heinemann.

Norris, C.M. 1999. Functional load abdominal training: part 1. *Journal of Bodywork and Movement Therapies* 3(3):150-58.

Norris, C.M., and Berry, S. 1998. Occurrence of common lumbar posture types in the student sporting population: an initial evaluation. *Sports, Exercise, and Injury* 4:15-18.

O'Sullivan, P.B.; Twomey, L.T.; and Allison, G.T. 1997. Evaluation of specific stabilizing exercise in the treatment of chronic low back pain with radiologic diagnosis of spondylolysis or spondylolisthesis. *Spine* 22:2959-67.

O'Sullivan, P.B.; Twomey, L.; and Allison, G.T. 1998. Altered abdominal muscle recruitment in patients with chronic back pain following a specific exercise intervention. *Journal of Orthopedic and Sports Physical Therapy* 27:114-24.

Oliver, J., and Middleditch, A. 1991. *Functional anatomy of the spine.* Oxford: Butterworth Heinemann.

Palastanga, N.; Field, D.; and Soames, R. 1994. *Anatomy and human movement.* 2d ed. Oxford: Butterworth Heinemann.

Panjabi, M.M. 1992. The stabilizing system of the spine. Part 1. Function, dysfunction, adaptation, and enhancement. *Journal of Spinal Disorders* 5:383-89.

Panjabi, M.M.; Abumi, K.; Duranceau, J.; and Oxland, T. 1989. Spinal stability and intersegmental muscle forces. A biomechanical model. *Spine* 14:194-200.

Panjabi, M.M.; Hult, J.E.; and White, A.A. 1987. Biomechanics studies in cadaveric spines. In *The lumbar spine and back pain,* ed. M.I.V. Jayson. Edinburgh: Churchill Livingstone.

Panjabi, M.M., and White, A.A. 1990. Physical properties and functional biomechanics of the spine. In *Clinical biomechanics of the spine,* ed. A.A. White and M.M. Panjabi. Philadelphia: Lippincott.

Paris, S.V. 1985. Physical signs of instability. *Spine* 10:277-79.

Parkkola, R.; Rytokoski, U.; and Kormano, M. 1993. Magnetic resonance imaging of the discs and trunk muscles in patients with chronic low back pain and healthy control subjects. *Spine* 18:830-36.

Parnianpour, M.; Nordin, M.; Kahanovitz, N.; and Frankel, V. 1988. The triaxial coupling of torque generation of trunk muscles during isometric exertions and the effect of fatiguing isoinertial movements on the motor output and movement patterns. *Spine* 13:982-92.

Pearcy, P.; Portek, I.; and Shepherd, J. 1984. Three dimensional X ray analysis of normal movement in the lumbar spine. *Spine* 9:294-97.

Perey, O. 1957. Fracture of the vertebral end plate in the lumbar spine. *Acta Orthop Scand* (Suppl) 25:1-101.

Pope, M.H., and Panjabi, M.M. 1985. Biomechanical definitions of instability. *Spine* 10:255-56.

Ricci, B.; Marchetti, M.; and Figura, F. 1981. Biomechanics of sit up exercises. *Medicine and Science in Sports and Exercise* 13:54-59.

Richardson, C.A. 1992. Muscle imbalance: principles of treatment and assessment. *Proceedings of the New Zealand Society of Physiotherapists Challenges Conference.* Christchurch, New Zealand.

Richardson, C.A., and Bullock, M.I. 1986. Changes in muscle activity during fast, alternating flexion-extension movements of the knee. *Scandinavian Journal of Rehabilitation Medicine* 18:51-58.

Richardson, C.A., and Hodges, P. 1996. New advances in exercise to rehabilitate spinal stabilisation. Course notes. University of Edinburgh.

Richardson, C.; Jull, G.; Toppenburg, R.; and Comerford, M. 1992. Techniques for active lumbar stabilisation for spinal protection: a pilot study. *Australian Journal of Physiotherapy* 38:105-12.

Richardson, C.A., and Sims, K. 1991. An inner range holding contraction: an objective measure of stabilising function of an antigravity muscle. *Proceedings of the World Confederation for Physical Therapy, 11th International Congress.* London.

Richardson, C.; Toppenberg, R.; and Jull, G. 1990. An initial evaluation of eight abdominal exercises for their ability to provide stabilisation for the lumbar spine. *Australian Journal of Physiotherapy* 36:6-11.

Risch, S.V.; Norvell, N.K.; Pollock, M.L.; Risch, E.D.; Langer, H.; Fulton, M.; Graves, J.E.; and Leggett, S.H. 1993. Lumbar strengthening in chronic low back pain patients. Physical and psychological benefits. *Spine* 18:232-38.

Roaf, R. 1960. A study of the mechanics of spinal injuries. *Journal of Bone and Joint Surgery* 42B:810-23.

Rockoff, S.F.; Sweet, E.; and Bleustein, J. 1969. The relative contribution of trabecular and cortical bone to the strength of human lumbar vertebrae. *Calcified Tissue Research* 3:163-75.

Saal, J.A. 1988. Rehabilitation of football players with lumbar spine injury. *Physician and Sportsmedicine* 16:61-67.

Saal, J.A. 1995. The pathophysiology of painful lumbar disorder. *Spine* 20:180-83.

Saal, J.A., and Saal, J.S. 1989. Nonoperative treatment of herniated lumbar intervertebral disc with radiculopathy. *Spine* 14:431-37.

Sahrmann, S.A. 1987. Posture and muscle imbalance: faulty lumbar-pelvic alignment and associated musculoskeletal pain syndromes. In *Postgraduate advances in physical therapy.* Berryvill, VA: Forum Medicum.

Sahrmann, S.A. 1990. Diagnosis and treatment of movement related pain syndromes associated with muscle and movement imbalances. Course notes. Washington University.

Silvermetz, M.A. 1990. Pathokinesiology of supine double leg lifts as an abdominal strengthener and suggested alternative exercises. *Athletic Training* 25:17-22.

Skall, F.H.; Manniche, C.; and Nielsen, C.J. 1994. Intensive back exercises 5 weeks after surgery of lumbar disk prolapse. A prospective randomized multicenter trial with a historical control group. *Ugeskr Laeger* 156:643-46.

Smith, R.L., and Brunolli, J. 1990. Shoulder kinesthesia after anterior glenohumeral joint dislocation. *Physical Therapy* 69:106-12.

Spitzer, W.O.; Le Blanc, F.E.; and Dupuis, M. 1987. Scientific approach to the assessment and management of activity related spinal disorders: a monograph for clinicians. Report of the Quebec Task Force on Spinal Disorders. *Spine* 12 (Suppl 7).

Sturesson, B.; Selvik, G.; and Uden, A. 1989. Movements of the sacroiliac joints. A roentgen stereophotogrammetric analysis. *Spine* 14:162-65.

Sugano, H., and Takeya, T. 1970. Measurement of body movement and its clinical application. *Japanese Journal of Physiology* 20:296-308.

Sullivan, M.S. 1997. Lifting and back pain. In *Physical therapy of the low back,* ed. L.T. Twomey and J.R. Taylor. Edinburgh: Churchill Livingstone.

Sullivan, P.E.; Markos, P.D.; and Minor, M.A.D. 1982. *An integrated approach to therapeutic exercise.* Reston, VA: Reston Publishing.

Swanepoel, M.W.; Adams, L.M.; and Smeathers, J.E. 1995. Human lumbar apophyseal joint damage and intervertebral disc degeneration. *Annals of the Rheumatic Diseases* 54:182-88.

Taylor, D.C.; Dalton, J.; Seaber, A.V.; and Garrett, W.E. 1990. The viscoelastic properties of muscle-tendon units. *American Journal of Sports Medicine* 18:300-09.

Taylor, J.R., and Twomey, L.T. 1986. Age changes in lumbar zygapophyseal joints. *Spine* 11:739-45.

Templeton, G.H.; Padalino, M.; and Manton, J. 1984. Influence of suspension hypokinesia on rat soleus muscle. *Journal of Applied Physiology* 56:278-86.

Thapa, P.B.; Gideon, P.; Brockman, K.G.; Fought, R.L.; and Ray, W.A. 1996. Clinical and biomechanical measures of balance as fall predictors in ambulatory nursing home residents. *Journal of Gerontology* 51:239-46.

Tkaczuk, H. 1968. Tensile properties of human lumbar longitudinal ligaments. *Acta Orthop Scand* 115 (Suppl).

Toppenburg, R.M., and Bullock, M.I. 1986. The interrelation of spinal curves, pelvic tilt and muscle lengths in the adolescent female. *Australian Journal of Physiotherapy* 32:6-12.

Travell, J.G., and Simmons, D.G. 1983. *Myofascial pain and dysfunction.* Baltimore: Williams & Wilkins.

Tropp, H.; Alaranta, H.; and Renstrom, P.A.F.H. 1993. Proprioception and coordination training in injury prevention. In *Sports injuries: basic principles of prevention and care.* IOC Medical Commission publication, ed. P.A.F.H. Renstrom. London: Blackwell Scientific.

Twomey, L.T., and Taylor, J.R. 1987. Lumbar posture, movement and mechanics. In *Physical therapy of the low back,* ed. L.T. Twomey. New York: Churchill Livingstone.

Twomey, L.T., and Taylor, J.R. 1994. Factors influencing ranges of movement in the spine. In *Physical therapy of the low back.* 2d ed., ed. L.T. Twomey and J.R. Taylor. Edinburgh: Churchill Livingstone.

Twomey, L.T.; Taylor, J.R.; and Oliver, M. 1988. Sustained flexion loading, rapid extension loading of the lumbar spine and the physical therapy of related injuries. *Physiotherapy Practice* 4:129-38.

Tye, J., and Brown, V. 1990. *Back pain—the ignored epidemic.* London: British Safety Council.

Tyldesley, B., and Grieve, J.I. 1989. *Muscles, nerves and movement: kinesiology in daily living.* Oxford: Blackwell Scientific.

Tyrrell, A.R.; Reilly, T.; and Troup, J.D.G. 1985. Circadian variation in stature and the effects of spinal loading. *Spine* 10:161-64.

Valencia, F.P., and Munro, R.R. 1985. An electromyographic study of the lumbar multifidus in man. *Electromyography and Clinical Neurophysiology* 25:205-21.

Vernon-Roberts, B. 1987. Pathology of intervertebral discs and apophyseal joints. In *The lumbar spine and back pain*, ed. M.I.V. Jayson. Edinburgh: Churchill Livingstone.

Vernon-Roberts, B. 1992. Age related and degenerative pathology of intervertebral discs and apophyseal joints. In *The lumbar spine and back pain*, ed. M.I.V. Jayson. Edinburgh: Churchill Livingstone.

Videman, T.; Nurminen, M.; and Troup, J.D.G. 1990. Lumbar spine pathology in cadaveric material in relation to history of back pain, occupation, and physical loading. *Spine* 15:728-40.

Vlaeyen, J.W.S.; Kole-Snijders, A.M.J.; Boeren, R.G.B.; and van Eek, H. 1995. Fear of movement/reinjury in chronic low back pain and its relation to behavioural performance. *Pain* 62:363-72.

Vleeming, A.; Mooney, V.; Snijders, C.J.; Dorman, T.A.; and Stoeckart, R. 1997. *Movement stability and low back pain.* New York: Churchill Livingstone.

Vleeming, A.; Pool-Goudzwaard, A.L.; and Stoeckart, R. 1995a. The posterior layer of the thoracolumbar fascia: its function in load transfer from spine to legs. *Spine* 20:753-58.

Vleeming, A.; Pool-Goudzwaard, A.L.; Stoeckart, R.; Wingerden, J.P.; and Snijders, C.J. 1995. The posterior layer of the thoracolumbar fascia: its function in load transfer from spine to legs. *Spine* 20:753-58.

Vleeming, A.; Stoeckart, R.; and Snijders, C. 1989. The sacrotuberous ligament: a conceptual approach to its dynamic role in stabilizing the sacroiliac joint. *Clinical Biomechanics* 4:201-03.

Vleeming, A.; Stoeckart, R.; Volkers, A.C.W.; and Snijders, C.J. 1990. Relation between form and function in the sacroiliac joint. *Spine* 15:130-32.

Waddell, G. 1987. A new clinical model for the treatment of low-back pain. *Spine* 12:632-44.

Waddell, G.; Feder, G.; and Lewis, M. 1997. Systematic reviews of bed rest and advice to stay active for acute low back pain. *British Journal of General Practice* 47:647-52.

Walker, M.L.; Rothstein, J.M.; Finucane, S.D.; and Lamb, R.L. 1987. Relationships between lumbar lordosis, pelvic tilt, and abdominal muscle performance. *Physical Therapy* 67:512-16.

Walters, C., and Partridge, M. 1957. Electromyographic study of the differential abdominal muscles during exercise. *American Journal of Physical Medicine* 36:259-68.

Watkins, J. 1999. *Structure and function of the musculoskeletal system.* Champaign, IL: Human Kinetics.

Watson, D.H. 1994. Cervical headache: an investigation of natural head posture and upper cervical flexor muscle performance. In *Grieve's modern manual therapy.* 2d ed., ed. J.D. Boyline and N. Palastanga. Edinburgh: Churchill Livingstone.

Watson, J. 1983. *An introduction for mechanics of human movement.* Lancaster, UK: MTP Press.

Weber, H. 1983. Lumbar disc herniation: a controlled prospective study with ten years of observation. *Spine* 8:131-38.

Webright, W.G.; Randolph, B.J.; and Perrin, D.H. 1997. Comparison of nonballistic active knee extension in neural slump position and static techniques on hamstring flexibility. *Journal of Orthopedic and Sports Physical Therapy* 26:7-13.

Weider, J. 1989. *Ultimate bodybuilding.* Chicago: Contemporary Books.

White, S.G., and Sahrmann, S.A. 1994. A movement system balance approach to management of musculoskeletal pain. In *Physical therapy of the cervical and thoracic spine*, ed. R. Grant. New York: Churchill Livingstone.

Wilke, H.J.; Wolf, S.; Claes, L.E.; Arand, M.; and Weisend, A. 1995. Stability increase of the lumbar spine with different muscle groups: a biomechanical in vitro study. *Spine* 20:192-98.

Willard, F.H. 1997. The muscular, ligamentous and neural structure of the low back and its relation to back pain. In *Movement stability and low back pain*, ed. A. Vleeming, V. Mooney, T. Dorman, C. Snijders, and R. Stoeckart. Edinburgh: Churchill Livingstone.

Williams, P.; Watt, P.; Bicik, V.; and Goldspink, G. 1986. Effect of stretch combined with electrical stimulation on the type of sarcomeres produced at the ends of muscle fibers. *Experimental Neurology* 93:500-09.

Williams, P.E. 1990. Use of intermittent stretch in the prevention of serial sarcomere loss in immobilised muscle. *Annals of the Rheumatic Diseases* 49:316-17.

Williams, P.E., and Goldspink, G. 1978. Changes in sarcomere length and physiological properties in immobilised muscle. *Journal of Anatomy* 127:459-68.

Yamamoto, I.; Panjabi, M.M.; Oxland, T.R.; and Crisco, J.J. 1990. The role of the iliolumbar ligament in the lumbosacral junction. *Spine* 15:1138-41.

Yang, K.H., and King, A.I. 1984. Mechanism of facet load transmission as a hypothesis for low back pain. *Spine* 9:557-65.

Yong-Hing, K.; Reilly, J.; and Kirkaldy-Willis, W.H. 1976. The ligamentum flavum. *Spine* 1:226-34.

Zetterberg, C.; Andersson, G.B.J.; and Schultz, A.B. 1987. The activity of individual trunk muscles during heavy physical loading. *Spine* 12:1035-40.

Zusman, M. 1998. Structure-oriented beliefs and disability due to back pain. *Australian Journal of Physiotherapy* 44:13-20.

Credits

From J.C. Griffin, 1998, *Client-centered exercise prescription* (Champaign, IL: Human Kinetics): **Figure 5.1 (page 95)** reprinted, by permission, from p. 176.

From J.A. Hides, C.A. Richardson, and G.A. Jull, 1996, "Multifidus muscle recovery is not automatic after resolution of acute, first-episode low back pain," *Spine* 21 (23): **Figure 3.5 (page 52)** reprinted, by permission, from pp. 2763-2769.

From National Strength and Conditioning Association, 1994, *Essentials of strength conditioning and training* (Champaign, IL: Human Kinetics): **Exercise figure, a-c, "Hang Clean" (Page 220)** adapted, by permission, from p. 394; **Exercise figure, a-c, "Power Clean" (page 221)** adapted, by permission, from p. 392; **Exercise figure, a-c, "Dead Lift" (page 222)** adapted, by permission, from p. 380.

From C. Norris, 1995, "Spinal stabilisation," *Physiotherapy Journal* 81 (3): **Exercise figure, a-c, "Assessing Muscle Balance in the Gluteus Maximus" (page 104)** reprinted, by permission, from p. 26.

From C. Norris, 1998, *Diagnosis and management*, 2d ed. (Oxford: Butterworth Heinemann): **Figure 2.12, a and b (page 30); Figure 2.14, a and b (page 34); Figure 2.16 (page 38)** reprinted from p. 18; **Exercise figure, a-d, "Knee Raising in Standing" (page 71); Exercise figure, a-d, "Assessing Lumbar-Pelvic Rhythm in Prone Kneeling" (page 72); Exercise figure, a and b, "The Hip Hinge Movement in Standing" (page 72); Exercise figure, a and b, "Recognizing False Hip Abduction" (Page 73)** reprinted from p. 167; **Figure 4.4 (page 91)** reprinted from p. 155; **Chapter 5 exercise descriptions; Figure 5.2 (page 95)** and **Figure 5.3 a (page 95)** reprinted from p. 145; **Figure 5.7 (page 101)** and **Figure 5.8 (page 101); Exercise figure, "Assessing Muscle Balance in the Iliopsoas" (page 103); Exercise figure, top right, "Assessing Muscle Balance in the Gluteus Maximus" (page 104); Exercise figure, "Assessing Muscle Balance in the Gluteus Medius" (page 105); Exercise figure, "Half Lunge" (page 114), Exercise figure, "Hip Hitch" (page 115), Exercise figure, "Active Knee Extension, Holding Thigh" (Page 116), Exercise figure, "Active Knee Extension, Pushing Against Thigh" (Page 116)** and **Exercise figure, "Tripod Stretch" (page 117)** reprinted from p. 175; **Figure 6.1, a and b (page 121)** reprinted from p. 176; **Figure 6.2 (page 122)** and **Figure 6.3 (page 125)** reprinted from p. 177; **Exercise figure, "Leg Lowering" (page 128); Exercise figure, "Bench Lying Pelvic Raise" (page 129)** and **Exercise figure, a, "Wall Bar Hanging Leg Raise" (page 130)** reprinted from p. 177; **Exercise figure, "Plyometric Flexion and Extension Using a Punching Bag" (page 226)** and **Exercise figure, "Leg Raise Throw (Page 227)** reprinted from p. 129. All reprinted by permission of Butterworth Heinemann Publishers, a division of Reed Educational & Professional Publishing Ltd.

From C.M. Norris, 1997, *Abdominal Training* (London: A & C Black): **Exercise figure, "Correction of Swayback Posture" (page 151)** and **Exercise figure, a and b, "Passive Back Extension in Lying Position" (page 156)** adapted, by permission, from p. 38. Illustrations by Jean Ashley.

From P.B. O'Sullivan, L.T. Twomey, and G.T. Allison, 1997, "Evaluation of specific stabilizing exercise in the treatment of chronic low back pain with radiological diagnosis of spondylolysis or spondylolisthesis," *Spine* 22 (24): **Figure 1.1 (page 7)** adapted, by permission, from pp. 2959-2967.

From C.A. Richardson and M.I. Bullock, 1986, "Changes in muscle activity during fast, alternating flexion-extension movements of the knee," *Scandinavian Journal of Rehabilitation Medicine* 18: **Figure 5.4 (page 98)** and **Figure 5.5 (page 98)**, reprinted, by permission, from pp. 51-58.

From J. Watkins, 1999, *Structure and function of the musculoskeletal system* (Champaign, IL: Human Kinetics): **Figure 2.1 (page 15)** reprinted from p. 61; **Figure 2.2 (page 15)** reprinted from p. 63; **Figure 2.5 (page 19)** reprinted from p. 145; **Figure 2.6 (page 19)** reprinted from p. 150.

Index

Figures and tables are indicated by the italicized letters t and f following the page number. Exercises and assessments have italicized page numbers.

A

abdominal hollowing: about 60; assessing 236; basic process 81; common errors 88-89; correct and incorrect positions 88; four-point kneeling 83; general considerations 81-82; importance 168; lying 85-86; with pelvic floor contractions 84; prone test using pressure biofeedback 105-106; standing 84; starting positions 82-86; teaching clients 81-89; teaching tips 86; two-point kneeling and sitting 85; with webbing belt 87f; in weight training 203

abdominal machine 212

abdominal muscles: activation in chronic low back pain 60f; coordination during spinal movement 60-62; deep abdominals anatomy 57-58; deep dissection illustration 58f; "doming" of abdominal wall 121; functions 58-60; intermediate dissection illustration 57f; in resisted actions 59; superficial abdominals anatomy 55-57

abdominal slide 188

abdominal training: current practice 120-124; modifications of traditional exercises 124-130

abdominal wall "doming" 121

ab roller exercises 130-132

active knee extension: holding thigh 116; pushing against thigh 116-117

active lumbar stability 12

active positioning reproduction 80-81

active stretching 111t, 112, 113

acute pain case history 242-244

Adams, M. 31

Adam's position 138

adipose tissue pad 22-23

advanced training qualifications 167-168

aerobic exercise 99

aging: chronic muscle tightness 237; compression of vertebral bodies 25; disc changes 28; facet joint cartilage 23; and ligaments 20; lumbar disc changes 28f; and posture 136; proteoglycan content 22; tissue overstretch 31

Allan, D.B. 6

American Academy of Orthopaedic Surgeons 134

anaerobic exercise 99

Andersson, E. 55

annulus fibrosis 20-21, 21f

anterior pelvic tilt 34f

anterolateral muscles 7

aponeurosis 45

approximate (verb), defined 45

arch mechanics 39f

arctan formula 142

arm fixation 123-124

arm lift in four-point kneeling 196-197

articulate, defined 17

articulating triad 14

assessments: heel slide maneuver using pressure biofeedback 106; hip hinge movement in standing 72-73; knee raising in standing 71; lumbar-pelvic rhythm in prone kneeling 72; muscle balance in gluteus maximus 104; muscle balance in gluteus medius 105; muscle balance in iliopsoas 103; Ober test 108-109; passive assessment of pelvic tilt 72; pelvic motion control in frontal plane 73; prone abdominal hollowing test using pressure biofeedback 105-106; recognizing false hip abduction 73-74; straight-leg raise test 109-110; Thomas test 107-108; tripod test 110

assisted pelvic tilt: from crook lying position 75-76; while sitting 75; while standing 74

atrophy 97

axial compression: of facet joints 28-29; of intervertebral discs 26-28; verterbal bodies 25-26

B

back care, in home 249f

back extension (frame) 209

back extension (machine) 208

back flattening 149-150

back muscles 52f

back pain: back stability exercises 234t; diagnostic triage 233; nonorganic causes 4-5; recurrence 3; scope of problem 3-4

back pain management: about 5-6; lumbar stabilization model 7-12; new model 6-7; traditional model 6

back stability assessment 236

back stability exercises 234t

Baechle, T.R. 214

balance boards 168-169, 183-186

ballistic stretching 111t, 112, 113

barbell lunge 218-219

Barrack, R.L. 199-200

basic crunch, ab roller 131

basic superman 190

bed rest 5, 234

behavioral factors 5

bench curl 127

bench lying pelvic raise 129

bending: erector spinae 37; sacroiliac joint 25; torsional stresses 27

bent knee sit-up 126

Biedermann, H.J. 51

blood flow, out of vertebral body 26

About the Author

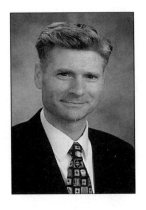

Christopher M. Norris, MSc, MCSP, has more than twenty years of experience as a physiotherapist and sport scientist. His specialty is exercise therapy. He is currently the director of Norris Associates in Manchester, UK.

An expert on back stability, Norris is the author of four books. One of his books on sports injuries is in its second edition and has been adopted by most physiotherapy schools in the United Kingdom. He has taught for the British Association of Sports Medicine on flexibility training and back rehabilitation. In addition to serving as a consultant to major companies, Norris also published the first-ever review of back stability in a series of articles in *Physiotherapy Journal*.

Norris is a member of the Chartered Society of Physiotherapy and the Society of Orthopaedic Medicine. He holds a certificate in occupational health physiotherapy, an advanced certificate in acupuncture, and a certificate in business administration.

He and his wife Hildegard live in the Peak District National Park. He enjoys hill walking and ju jitsu.